# BIOCHEMICAL AND PHARMACOLOGICAL ROLES OF ADENOSYLMETHIONINE AND THE CENTRAL NERVOUS SYSTEM

# BIOCHEMICAL AND PHARMACOLOGICAL ROLES OF ADENOSYLMETHIONINE AND THE CENTRAL NERVOUS SYSTEM

Proceedings of an International Round Table on
Adenosylmethionine and the Central Nervous System
Naples, Italy, May 1978

Editors

**VINCENZO ZAPPIA**

University of Naples
Naples, Italy

**EARL USDIN**

National Institute of Mental Health
Rockville, Maryland, USA

**FRANCESCO SALVATORE**

University of Naples
Naples, Italy

# PERGAMON PRESS

OXFORD · NEW YORK · TORONTO · SYDNEY · PARIS · FRANKFURT

| U.K. | Pergamon Press Ltd., Headington Hill Hall, Oxford OX3 0BW, England |
| U.S.A. | Pergamon Press Inc., Maxwell House, Fairview Park, Elmsford, New York 10523, U.S.A. |
| CANADA | Pergamon of Canada, Suite 104, 150 Consumers Road, Willowdale, Ontario M2J 1P9, Canada |
| AUSTRALIA | Pergamon Press (Aust.) Pty. Ltd., P.O. Box 544, Potts Point, N.S.W. 2011, Australia |
| FRANCE | Pergamon Press SARL, 24 rue des Ecoles, 75240 Paris, Cedex 05, France |
| FEDERAL REPUBLIC OF GERMANY | Pergamon Press GmbH, 6242 Kronberg-Taunus, Pferdstrasse 1, Federal Republic of Germany |

First edition 1979

**British Library Cataloguing in Publication Data**

Adenosylmethionine and the Central Nervous System (conference), Naples, 1978
Biochemical and pharmacological roles of adenosylmethionine and the central nervous system.
1. Neurochemistry
2. Central nervous system. 3. Adenosylmethionine
I. Title II. Zappia, Vincenzo III. Usdin, Earl
IV. Salvatore, Francesco
612'.8     QP356.3     79-40691
ISBN 0-08-024929-9

In order to make this volume available as economically and as rapidly as possible the authors' typescripts have been reproduced in their original forms. This method unfortunately has its typographical limitations but it is hoped that they in no way distract the reader.

Printed and bound at William Clowes & Sons Limited
Beccles and London

# Contents

# Preface

This volume contains thirteen contributions by experts on the biochemical and pharmacological roles of S-adenosylmethionine (SAM), with particular emphasis on the functions of this compound in the central nervous system (CNS). The reports were presented at a round-table meeting held in Naples (Italy) on May 2, 1978. This specialized meeting was organized in response to the rapid expansion of this field. The organizers regretted that it was impossible to accomodate other outstanding investigators within the program of the meeting and hope this volume will allow others interested in the role of SAM in the CNS to profit from the presentations.

The Editors wish to express their thanks to the speakers, the discussants, the section chairmen and to the other participants. The meeting was sponsored by the "Accademia di Scienze Mediche di Napoli" and the Editors wish to express their appreciation to Professor L. Donatelli, Secretary of the Accademia, for his cooperation. They also acknowledge the generous hospitality at the Villa Pignatelli of the "Sovraintendenza delle Belle Arti di Napoli" as well as the support received from Dr. L. Camozzi of the Bio-Research Laboratories and from the "Azienda di Soggioinoe Cura di Napoli".

Meetings on SAM were initiated in 1964 when Drs. Shapiro and Schlenk organized the first one at the Argonne National Laboratory in the United States. Then after a rather long break two meetings followed in close succession: one at Gif-sur-Yvette (France), organized by Drs. Lederer and Cantoni in 1973, and one in 1974 in Rome (Italy) through the efforts of Drs. Salvatore, Borek, Zappia, Williams-Ashman and Schlenk. In addition to the Naples meeting on SAM in the CNS in 1978, there is also scheduled a Conference on Transmethylation for October in Bethesda (U.S.A.), organized by Usdin, Borchardt and Creveling.

The reports in this volume include an introductory review on some novel biochemical aspects of SAM and seven papers concerned with several chemical and biochemical properties of this molecule, with special reference to its roles in the CNS. The five papers which follow deal with pharmacological aspects of SAM within the CNS and also with attempted clinical use of this compound. The clinical utility of SAM would be of remarkable interest, if it can be confirmed by further studies.

The Editors would like to recall that the trial of the topics of this symposium was opened by the studies of Dr. Julius Axelrod: the discovery in the CNS of methylating enzymes which metabolize catecholamines and other aromatic compounds. The trial continues to be lighted today by his studies on protein methylation and the role of SAM in the excitation-secretion coupling at the level of the outer surface of the chromaffin vesicle. Thus, we dedicate this volume to the work of Julius Axelrod.

*Vincenzo Zappia*
*Earl Usdin*
*Francesco Salvatore*

# Abbreviations

ACTH = adrenocorticotrophic hormone
Ado-Hcy cf SAH
ADO-MET cf SAM
AP = anterior pituitary
asDMArg = $N^G,N^G$-di(asymmetric)arginine
ATP = adenosine 5'-triphosphate
BBB = blood-brain barrier
CEEG = computerized EEG
$CH_3FH_4$ = $N^5$-methyltetrahydrofolate
CNS = central nervous system
COMT = catechol 0-methyltransferase
CPT = protein carboxy transferase
CPZ = chlorpromazine
DBN = 2,3,4,6,7,8-hexahydro-pyrrolo
[1,2-a]pyrimidine
deca SAM = decarboxylated SAM = S-adenosyl-
5'-methylthiopropylamine
DMT = N,N-dimethyltryptamine
DNA = deoxyribonucleic acid
DOPA = Dopa = dopa = 3,4-dihydroxyphenyl-
alanine
dTMP = deoxythymidine monophosphate
dUMP = deoxyuridine monophosphate
E. coli = Escherichia coli
EEG = electroencephalograph
β-EP = β-endorphin
FAD = favin adenine dinucleotide
$FH_4$ = tetrahydrofolate
FSH = follicle stimulating hormone
GH = growth hormone
GLC = gas-liquid chromatography
GTP = guanosine-5'-triphosphate
H = histamine
HHPRLA = hypothalamic-hypophyseal-prolac-
tin axis
5-HIAA = HIAA = 5-hydroxyindoleactic acid
HIF = hypothalamic inhibitory factor
HIMT cf HIOMT
HIOMT = hydroxyindole 0-methyltransferase
HMT = histamine N-methyltransferase
HNMT - cf HMT
HPLC = high (performance or pressure)
liquid chromatography
HRF = hypothalamic releasing factor
HRS = Hamilton Rating Scale (for Depression)

5-HT = serotonin
GABA = γ-aminobutyric acid
HnRNP = heterogenous nuclear ribonucleo-
protein
HVA = homovanillic acid
INMT = indoleamine N-methyltransferase
LH = luteinizine hormone
LSD = lysergic acid diethylamide
MAO = monoamine oxidase
ME = median eminence
$m^5FH_4$ = $N^5$-methyltetrahydrofolate
MHPG-SO$_4$ = 3-methoxy-4-hydroxyphenyl-
glycol sulfate
M.I.T. = MIT = Massachusetts Insti-
tute of Technology
MMArg = $N^G$-(mono)methylarginine
MTA = methylthioadenosine
MTHF = methyltetrahydrofolate
NADPH = NAD(P)H = reduced **triphospho-
pyridine nucleotide**
NE = norepinephrine
NEA = neuro-endocrine axis
NIMH = (U.S.) National Institute of
Mental Health
NMT = N-methyltryptamine
nor$_1$CPZ = N-demethyl CPZ
nor$_2$CPZ = di-N-demethyl CPZ
PCMB = p-chloromercuribenzoic acid
Pi = inorganic phosphate
PIF = prolactin inhibitory factor
PLP = pyridoxal-5'-phosphate
PNMT = phenylethanolamine N-methyl-
transferase
PRL = prolactin
RNA = ribonucleic acid
SAH = S-adenosylhomocysteine
SAM = S-adenosylmethionine
sDMArg = $N^G,N'^G$-di(symmetric)arginine
SMM = S-methylmethionine
TIDA = tubero-infundibular system
TLC = thin-layer chromatography
tRNA = transfer RNA
TSH = thyrotropin stimulating hormone
VMA = vanillylmandelic acid

# Contributors

Algeri, Sergio
Institute of Pharmacological Research
"Mario Negri", Via Eritrea 62
20157 Milano, Italy

Amati, Amato
Department of Psychiatry
Ist Medical School
University of Naples
80100 Napoli, Italy

Baldessarini, Ross J.
Mailman Laboratories for
  Psychiatric Research
McLean Division of
Massachusetts General Hospital
Belmont, Massachusetts 20178 USA

Benzi, Gianni
Institute of Pharmacology
University of Pavia
Facolta di Scienze
27100 Pavia, Italy

Cacciapuoti, Giovanna
Department of Biochemistry
Ist Medical School
University of Naples
Via Costantinopoli 16
80138 Napoli, Italy

Catto, Emilia
Institute of Pharmacological Research
"Mario Negri" Via Eritrea 62
20157 Milano, Italy

Celani, Tiziana
Department of Psychiatry
Ist Medical School
University of Naples
80100 Napoli, Italy

Clementi, Giuseppe
Department of Pharmacology
School of Medicine
University of Catania
95125 Catania, Italy

Curcio, Maria
Institute of Pharmacological Research
"Mario Negri", Via Eritrea 62
20157 Milano, Italy

Della Pietra, Gennaro
Department of Biochemistry
Ist Medical School
University of Naples
Via Costantinopoli 16
80138 Napoli, Italy

Del Vecchio, Mario
Department of Psychiatry
Ist Medical School
University of Naples
80100 Napoli, Italy

Eloranta, Terho E.
Department of Biochemistry
University of Kuopio
P.O.B. 138
SF-70101
Kuopio 10, Finland

Esposito, Carla
Department of Biochemistry
Ist Medical School
University of Naples
Via Costantinopoli 16
80138 Napoli, Italy

Famiglietti, Luciana A.
Department of Psychiatry
Ist Medical School
University of Naples
80100 Napoli, Italy

Fiecchi, Alberto
Department of Chemistry
Medical School
University of Milan
Via Saldini, 50
20133 Milano, Italy

Galletti, Patrizia
Department of Biochemistry
Ist Medical School
University of Naples
Via Costantinopoli, 16
80138 Napoli, Italy

Kemali, Dargut
Department of Psychiatry
Ist Medical School
University of Naples
80100 Napoli, Italy

Kim, Sangduk
Fels Research Institute
Temple University School of Medicine
Philadelphia, Pennsylvania 19140, USA

Lipinski, Joseph F.
Department of Psychiatry
Harvard Medical School
Boston, Massachusetts, USA

Mason, Robert J.
Department of Biochemistry
University of Leeds
9 Hyde Terrace
Leeds LS 2 9LS, England

Paik, Woon Ki
Fels Research Institute
Temple University School of Medicine
Philadelphia, Pennsylvania 19140, USA

Pearson, Andrew G.M.
Department of Biochemistry
University of Leeds
9 Hyde Terrace
Leeds LS2 9LS, England

Ponzio, Franca
Institute of Pharmacological Research
"Mario Negri", Via Eritrea 62
20157 Milano, Italy

Porcelli, Marina
Department of Biochemistry
Ist Medical School
University of Naples
Via Costantinopoli 16
80138 Napoli, Italy

Porta, Raffaele
Department of Biochemistry
Ist Medical School
University of Naples
Via Costantinopoli 16
80138 Napoli, Italy

Prato, Agata
Department of Pharmacology
School of Medicine
University of Catania
Catania, Italy

Ragusa, Nicola
Department of Pharmacology
School of Medicine
University of Catania
Catania, Italy

Rizza, Victor
Department of Pharmacology
School of Medicine
University of Catania
Catania, Italy

Salvatore, Francesco
Department of Biochemistry
2nd Medical School
University of Naples
Via Sergio Pansini 5
80131 Napoli, Italy

Scapagnini, Umberto
Department of Pharmacology
School of Medicine
University of Catania
Catania, Italy

Schatz, Robert A.
Laboratory of Neurochemistry
Mental Health Research Institute
University of Michigan Medical Center
Ann Arbor, Michigan 48109, USA

Sellinger, Otto Z.
Laboratory of Neurochemistry
Mental Health Research Institute
University of Michigan Medical Center
Ann Arbor, Michigan 48109, USA

Stramentinoli, Giorgio
Department of Biochemistry
Bio-Research Co.
20060 Liscate (Milan), Italy

Turner, Anthony J.
Department of Biochemistry
University of Leeds
9 Hyde Terrace
Leeds LS2 9LS, England

Usdin, Earl
Psychopharmacology Research Branch
National Institute of Mental Health
Rockville, Maryland 20857, USA

Vacca, Lucio
Department of Psychiatry
Ist Medical School
University of Naples
80100 Napoli, Italy

Wurtman, Richard J.
Laboratory of Neuroendocrine Regulation
Massachusetts Institute of Technology
Cambridge, Massachusetts, 02139, USA

Zappia, Vincenzo
Department of Biochemistry
Ist Medical School
University of Naples
Via Costantinopoli 16
80138 Napoli, Italy

# Novel Aspects in the Biochemistry of Adenosylmethionine and Related Sulfur Compounds

**Vincenzo Zappia, Francesco Salvatore, Marina Porcelli and Giovanna Cacciapuoti**

Departments of Biochemistry, 1st and 2nd Medical School, University of Naples, Naples, Italy

In recent years, since the Symposium on "The Biochemistry of Adenosylmethionine" held in Rome in 1974 (1), several new metabolic functions have been assigned to this important and widely occurring sulfonium compound. The number of enzymatic reactions in which it functions either as substrate or as modulator has signif- icantly increased: few other molecules are indeed involved in so many different types of reactions within the cell. The only other sulfonium compound detectable in mammalian tissues is S-adenosyl-(5')-3-methylthiopropylamine, i.e., decarboxy- lated adenosylmethionine; the biological roles of the two compounds are summarized in Table 1.

Table 1    BIOLOGICAL ROLES OF S-ADENOSYLMETHIONINE (I) AND ITS
DECARBOXYLATED PRODUCT (II)

- DONOR OF METHYL GROUP IN A WIDE VARIETY OF TRANSMETHYLATION REACTIONS (I).

- DONOR OF PROPYLAMINE MOIETY IN THE BIOSYNTHESIS OF SPERMIDINE, SYM-NOR-SPERMIDINE, SPERMINE AND SYM-NOR-SPERMINE (II).

- SUBSTRATE OF A SPECIFIC LYASE WHICH CONVERTS THE MOLECULE INTO 5'-METHYL-THIOADENOSINE AND HOMOSERINE (I).

- DONOR OF THE AMINOBUTYRYL SIDE CHAIN TO tRNA (I).

- DONOR OF THE SIDE CHAIN AMINO GROUP IN BIOTIN BIOSYNTHESIS (I).

- ADENOSYL DONOR (I).

- ACTIVATOR OF LYSINE-2,3-AMINO MUTASE, THREONINE SYNTHETASE, PYRUVATE-FORMATE-LYASE AND $N^5$ -METHYLTETRAHYDROFOLATE-HOMOCYSTEINE METHYL-TRANSFERASE (I).

- INHIBITOR OF RIBONUCLEASE H, METHYLENE TETRAHYDROFOLIC REDUCTASE AND ETHANOLAMINEPHOSPHATE CYTIDYLTRANSFERASE (I).

- REQUIRED FOR BACTERIAL CHEMOTAXIS (I).

- REQUIRED IN THE RESTRICTION AND MODIFICATION SYSTEM OF DNA IN PRO-KARYOTES AND EUKARYOTES (I).

1

## TRANSMETHYLATION REACTIONS

Transmethylation may be considered as the oldest example of biochemical group transfer and represents by far the largest and most widely studied group of alkyl transfer reactions (2).  In mammalian systems adenosylmethionine (SAM) is the most versatile methyl donor, while $N^5$-methyltetrahydrofolic acid (3), methylcobalamin (4) and betaine (5), are involved in transmethylations only in a few instances.

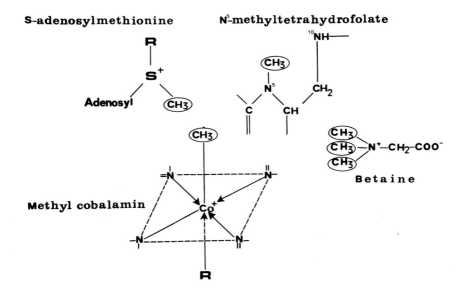

Fig. 1  Schematic representation of the biological methyl donors in mammalian systems

Fig. 1 gives a schematic representation of these molecules; the methyl group is bound respectively: to the sulfur atom in the onium configuration in SAM, to the trivalent nitrogen in the folic acid derivative, to the nitrogen in the ammonium form in betaine, and to the cobalt ion coordinated by four nitrogen atoms in the cobalamine derivative.  Whether the 5-N of methyltetrahydrofolate is quaternized (6) similarly to the nitrogen of betaine is matter of investigation.  The non-polar environment of the enzyme active site could facilitate such a conformation.

The chemical variety of acceptors of the methyl group from SAM is strikingly high: the attachment of the methyl group to the nitrogen atom is perhaps the most extensively studied, but sulfur, oxygen and carbon are also binding sites.  As far as the central nervous system (CNS) is concerned, methyl transfer reactions are often involved in the metabolism of several neuromediators and, in many instances, the methylated products possess psychotomimetic properties (7). All the reactions listed in Table 2 have been found to be operative in the CNS.

Table 2    METHYL TRANSFER REACTIONS IN CENTRAL NERVOUS SYSTEM

| ENZYME | TYPE OF BOND FORMED | EXAMPLES OF SUBSTRATES |
|---|---|---|
| COMT | O-CH$_3$ | NOR - ADRENALINE, ADRENALINE, DOPAMINE, L - DOPA, 3,4 - DIHYDROXY-MANDELIC ACID, 2 - HYDROXY-ESTRADIOL, ASCORBIC ACID. |
| HIOMT | | ACETYLSEROTONIN, SEROTONIN, 5 - HYDROXY - - INDOLE, BUFOTENINE |
| PROTEIN CARBOXYMETHYLASE | | LH, FSH, ACTH, GH, NEUROPHYSIN, TSH |
| HMT | N-CH$_3$ | HISTAMINE |
| PNMT | | NOR - ADRENALINE, METANEPHRINE, OCTOPA MINE, PHENYLETHANOLAMINE |
| NON SPECIFIC N - METHYLTRANSFERASE | | SEROTONIN, TRYPTAMINE, N - METHYLTRYP= TAMINE |
| PROTEIN - LYSINE METHYLASE | | HYSTONES |
| NUCLEIC ACID METHYLTRANSFERASES | { N-CH$_3$ O-CH$_3$ C-CH$_3$ | RNA AND DNA |

Besides the two most widely studied enzymes, namely catechol–methyl–transferase and hydroxyindole–methyltransferase, which are discussed in detail in this volume, the methylation of specific lysyl residues of histones in rat brain nuclei has been investigated by several laboratories (8–12); its regulatory significance with respect to gene expression is still a matter of speculation. Furthermore, the specific activity of histone methyltransferase has been found to be significantly higher in neuronal populations than in oligodendroglia nuclei (11).

It is interesting to note that one of the major endogenous substrates for protein carboxyl methyltransferase in posterior pituitary gland is the hormone binding protein, neurophysin (13). Fig. 2 shows the effect of vasopressin on the kinetics of methylation of neurophysin: the hormone increases the rate of methylation, thus suggesting that the methylation site and the hormone binding site are different (13). The possible regulatory significance of this effect deserves further investigation.

The short half–life of the carboxy–methyl group in proteins makes protein methylation a good candidate for a regulatory process, methanol being the product of demethylation (7). Very recently methylated catecholamines have also been described as

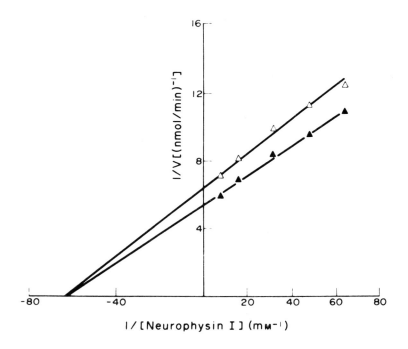

Fig. 2  Effect of vasopressin on neurophysin methylation.  Double re-
        ciprocal plot of methylation rates vs. neurophysin concentra-
        tion.  SAM concentration = 10 µM (△):  control (no hormone
        added: (▲).

demethylated in erythrocytes by an enzyme system which produces methanol (14).  The
search for the occurence of such enzyme in the CNS would be of extreme interest.

It is well known that several anterior pituitary polypeptides with hormonal activity are also methylated by carboxyl protein methylase; e.g., β-lipotropin, a
precursor of β-endorphin, has been reported to be methylated at a much higher rate
than β-endorphin (15,16).  It is tempting to speculate that methylation of the
polypeptide affects the processing of this class of hormones.

Bacterial chemotaxis is also related to methyl esterification of membrane protein,
which, in turn, affects response to chemoattractants (17,18).  Also in mammalian
systems, such as neutrophils which possess chemotactic responsiveness, methyl
esterification plays a critical role as a signal for leukocyte motion (19).

Methylation of nucleic acids at various base and sugar moieties appears to be involved in a variety of biological regulatory mechanisms, most of which are still
far from being understood at the molecular level.  Several reviews extensively
summarize emerging concepts in this field; we refer to these for detailed discus-

sion (20-24). We would only mention in this context that modification and restriction systems in bacterial and viral DNAs have been extensively studied and widely used as tools in genetic engineering (25-26). In fact methylation of DNA is most frequently a prerequisite for splitting the polynucleotide chain at very specific sites.

Monomethylation of the $N^6$-amino group of specific adenine residues in bacterial and viral DNAs has found particular attention (27,28), since it appears to be the first step for further methylation or restriction at the polynucleotide chain. Most likely the presence of the methyl group is essential for enzyme recognition as such. Alternatively, methylation may induce a change in the secondary structure and/or in the stability of the nucleic acid, which in turn could function as a partial determinant of specificity. Along this line, recent experiments (29) with poly (A-T) show that $N^6$-monomethylation, though not sufficient to produce open structures or base mismatching, makes such changes more probable to occur. Some possible conformations of methylated poly-d(A-T) are reported in Fig. 3 (see 29).

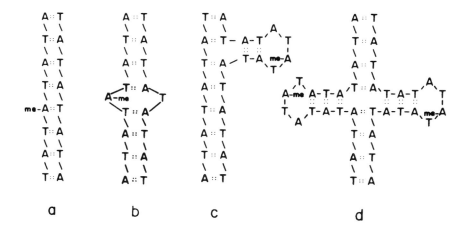

Fig. 3. Proposed conformations of methylated poly-d(A-T) (from Engel and von Hippel, 29)

tRNA and DNA methylases have been also found associated with Rous sarcoma virus particles (30-32); their significance in relation to the biology of virus infection and/or transformation still deserves further investigation.

POLYAMINE BIOSYNTHESIS AND UNUSUAL BIOCHEMICAL ROLES OF ADENOSYLMETHIONINE

The role of SAM as a precursor of polyamines is well known. Decarboxylated SAM is
the only biological donor, so far recognized, of the propylamine moiety in the
biosynthesis of polyamines.

Recent data from our laboratory demonstrate that decarboxylated SAM is also the
precursor of the newly described polyamines sym-nor-spermidine and sym-nor-spermine

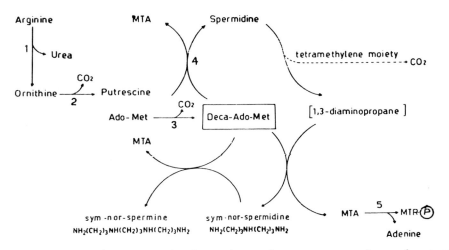

Fig. 4.   Biosynthetic pathway of sym-nor-spermine and sym-nor-spermidine
          (from De Rosa et al., 36).

(see Fig. 4): two moles of this sulfonium compound are required for the biosynthesis of sym-nor-spermidine and three moles for the biosynthesis of sym-nor-spermine (35-36). The steps in the biosynthetic pathway are unusual, since the carbon
skeleton of the new polyamines derives entirely from S-adenosyl-(5')3-methylthio-
propylamine. The occurrence of these symmetrical polyamines has been reported in
thermophylic bacteria (36) and in several arthropods (37). So far, the function of
decarboxylated SAM has been limited only to polyamines biosynthesis, though the
possibility of propylamino transfer to other acceptors, e.g., proteins, nucleic
acids, etc., has not yet been explored.

The observation that decarboxylated SAM is much more stable at elevated tempera-
tures and acid pH than its parent compound, allowed the development of new methods
of preparation and analysis of the molecule (38). Furthermore, the different behavior of the two molecules, with respect to the cleavage of the bond between the
sulfur and the carbon chain, presumably involves an intramolecular nucleophilic

attack of the carboxyl group of SAM on carbon atom 4 of the amino acid chain (2, 38).

The same reaction mechanism is operative in the enzymatic cleavage of the molecule into homoserine and methylthioadenosine, catalyzed by SAM lyase (see 39 and Table 1). The enzyme has been also detected in mammalian tissues (40-42); in rat liver the apparent $K_m$ for SAM corresponds to its cellular concentration, thus suggesting for this enzyme a possible regulatory role for cellular SAM concentration (40).

Another type of reaction (listed in Table 1) concerns the transfer of the unmodified amino acid side chain of SAM to the uridine nitrogen of tRNA, and represents one of the so-called nucleoside hypermodifications occurring in the maturation of tRNA (43, 44). The modified uridine, i.e., 3-(3-amino-3-carboxypropyl)-uridine, has been detected in bacterial and in mammalian tRNA, and its biological significance is probably related to the stabilization of the three-dimensional structure of the polynucleotide (44).

SAM may also undergo a transamination reaction in the pathway of biotin biosynthesis in E. coli (45-46). The reaction, catalyzed by diaminopelargonic acid aminotransferase, is illustrated in Fig. 5. The enzyme appears to be highly specific for

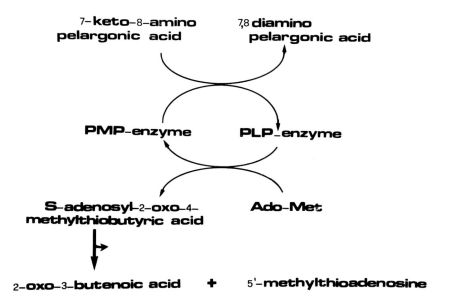

Fig. 5   Role of SAM in a transamination reaction in the pathway of biotin biosynthesis (from Stoner and Eisenberg, 46).

SAM, in fact S-adenosylethionine. S-adenosyl-homocysteine, S-methylmethionine and methionine were unable to transaminate with 7-keto-8-aminopelargonic acid.  It has been purified 1,000-fold from regulatory mutants of E. coli, derepressed for the enzymes of the biotin operon.  The co-enzymatic role of pyridoxal-5'-phosphate has been demonstrated, and the cofactor can be resolved from the enzyme after incubation with SAM (46).

The role of SAM as an adenosyl donor was postulated by Cantoni (47) on the basis of the equivalence of the three bonds around the sulfonium pole: the crystallo-graphic studies performed by Del Re et al. (48) on S-methylmethionine confirmed that the sulfonium group is pyramidal and that the three bond-lengths and angles around the sulfur are nearly equal.  The adenosylating function of SAM has been proposed in three instances: (i) in the reversal of the SAM synthetase reaction (49), (ii) in the pyruvate-formate lyase reaction (50), and (iii) in the lysine amino-mutase reaction (51).  The conversion of the inactive form of pyruvate-formate lyase into the catalytically active enzyme is accomplished by a "converter" enzyme, requiring SAM (50).  During the activation, the sulfonium compound is reductively processed into methionine, adenine and 5-deoxyribose and a transient adenosylation of the converter enzyme has been proposed (50).  A similar mechanism of protein adenosylation has been suggested for lysine mutase (51).  This enzyme is composed of four regulatory subunits which bind SAM and two catalytic subunits, as indicated in the scheme of Fig. 6.

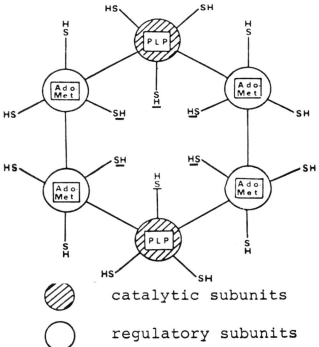

Fig. 6  Proposed structure of lysine mutase

The number of reactions where SAM exerts a regulatory role, either as a positive or as a negative effector, has significantly increased in recent years; some of them are listed in Table 1. The methylation of the enzyme molecule has been proposed as a mechanism of control of ethanolaminephosphate cytidyl-transferase activity (52); the methylation of the protein probably occurs through a non-enzymatic reaction, since S-adenosylhomocysteine, a typical inhibitor of methyltransferases does not modify the effect of SAM. The same mechanism has been proposed to explain the irreversible inactivation of calf thymus ribonuclease H exerted by SAM (53,54). The inhibition operated by the sulfonium compound on methylene-tetrahydrofolic reductase is extensively discussed elsewhere in this book (see Turner et al., 55).

METABOLIC PATHWAYS RELATED TO ADENOSINE-SULFUR COMPOUNDS

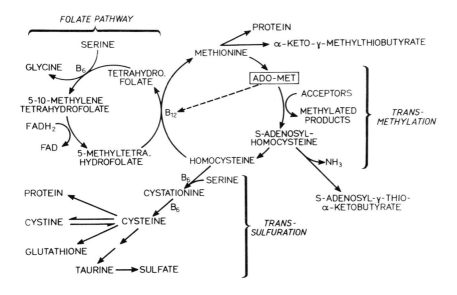

Fig. 7  Metabolic relationships among transmethylation, transsulfuration and the folate cycle.

In Fig. 7 are summarized the metabolic relationships among transmethylation, transsulfuration and the folate cycle. Via transmethylation, SAM is converted into adenosylhomocysteine, which in turn is a powerful inhibitor of all the methyl transfer reactions so far investigated. The adenosylhomocysteine degrading enzymes, namely L-amino acid oxidase (56) and a specific hydrolase (57), play, therefore, an indirect regulatory role on methyl transfer. Although the equilibrium of the hydrolytic reaction lies far in the direction of condensation, adenosylhomocysteine readily undergoes hydrolysis since the products are enzymatically removed. Adenosine is rapidly converted into inosine, hypoxanthine, xanthine and excreted as uric acid (58, see Fig. 8), while homocysteine is metabolized by two competing systems:

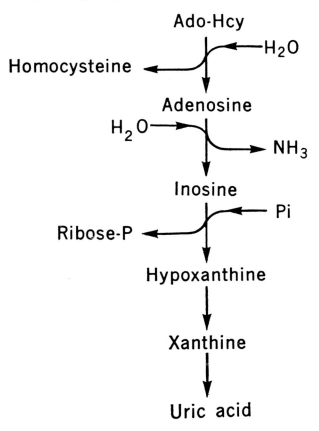

Fig. 8  Pathway of degradation of adenosylhomocysteine to uric acid in rat liver (from Cortese et al., 58).

the trans-sulfuration pathway leading to cysteine, and the so called "sulfur conservation cycle" connecting with the folate pathway.

Fig. 9 illustrates the three metabolic pathways related to SAM metabolism and not reported in the scheme of Fig. 7: the reactions from 1 to 3 lead to 5'methylthioadenosine as a common metabolic product. Methylthioadenosine nucleosidase is the main enzyme related to the degradation of this thioether; the reaction (pathway 4, Fig. 9) involves in the mammalian system the phosphorolytic cleavage of methylthioadenosine into methylthioribose-1-phosphate and adenine (59,60).

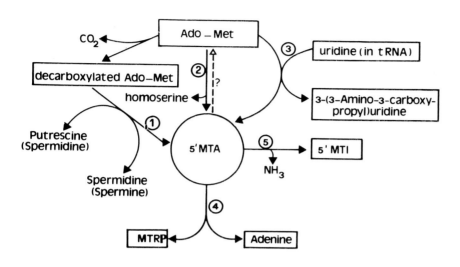

Fig. 9   Biosynthetic pathways of methylthioadenosine from SAM (from
        Cacciapuoti et al., 59).

TRANSPORT OF ADENOSYLMETHIONINE

Despite the numerous biological roles of SAM, the mechanism of transport of this
positively charged molecule in mammalian cells has been investigated only recently.
An active transport system with high affinity towards SAM has been described in
yeast cells (61,62), which accumulate very peculiarly the sulfonium compound into
the vacuoles (63):  mutants lacking this transport system have also been isolated
(61).   The incorporation of SAM by pancreas isolated cells (64), as well as by
rabbit erythrocytes (65), has also been investigated.   Fig. 10 shows the uptake of
several thioethers and sulfonium compounds by isolated and perfused rat liver (66).
The thioethers methionine and methylthioadenosine are incorporated at a higher
rate than the three sulfonium compounds.   The positively charged sulfonium probably limits the passage of the molecule into the cells: this is particularly evident
when the incorporation of methylthioadenosine is compared to that of dimethylthio-

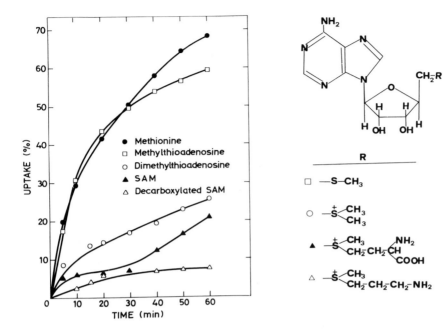

Fig. 10  Uptake of SAM and related sulfur compounds by isolated
and perfused rat liver (from Zappia <u>et al</u>., 66).

adenosine, two molecules mainly differing from each other in the net charge.  The
existence of a high-affinity permease, specific for thioethers, and a low-affinity
system, specific for sulfonium compounds, has been postulated (66).  The transport
system for SAM shows saturation kinetics, with an apparent $K_m$ of 60μM, and is en-
ergy-dependent, as demonstrated by the inhibition by 2,4-dinitrophenol.  The cellular
uptake of SAM has also been investigated in isolated rat hepatocytes and two distinct binding sites have been proposed (67).

A non-specific SAM binding protein, stimulating phosphatidylethanolamine and tRNA
methylation, has been recently purified from rat liver by Smith (68).  Whether this
protein is also involved in SAM transport deserves further investigation.


ACKNOWLEDGMENTS

The work performed in the laboratory of the authors has been partially supported
by CNR (Italy), through grants to V. Zappia (n. 77.01544.04) and F. Salvatore
(n. 77.01486.04 and n. 77.01559.65).

## REFERENCES

1. Salvatore, F., Borek E., Zappia V., Williams-Ashman H.G. and Schlenk, F., _The Biochemistry of Adenosylmethionine_, Columbia University Press, New York (1977).

2. Schlenk, F., in _Progress in the Chemistry of Organic Natural Products_, Zeichmeister, L., Ed., Springer - Verlag, Berlin, 23, 61 (1965).

3. Taylor, R.T. and Weissbach, H. in _The Enzymes_, Boyer, P.D., Ed., Academic Press, New York, 9, 121 (1973).

4. Lexmond, T.M., de Haan, F.A.M. and Frissel, M.J., _Neth. J. Agric. Sci._, 24, 79 (1976).

5. Mudd, S.H. and Levy, H.L., in _The Metabolic Basis of Inherited Disease_, Stanbury, J.B., Winegarden, J.B., Fredrikson, D.S., Eds., 4th Edition, 458 (1978).

6. Cantoni, G.L., _Ann. Rev. Biochem._, 44, 435 (1975).

7. Axelrod, J., in _The Biochemistry of Adenosylmethionine_, Salvatore F., Borek, E., Zappia, V., Williams-Ashman, H.G. and Schlenk, F., Eds., Columbia University Press, New York, 539 (1977).

8. Paik, W.K. and Kim, S., _Biochim. Biophys. Acta_, 313, 181 (1973).

9. Wallwork, J.C., Quick, D.P. and Duerre, J.A., _J. Biol. Chem._, 252, 5977 (1977).

10. Duerre, J.A., Wallwork, J.C., Quick, D.P. and Ford, K.M., _J. Biol. Chem._, 252. 5981 (1977).

11. Lee, N.M. and Loh, H.H., _J. Neurochem._, 29, 547 (1977).

12. Moller, M.L., Miller, H.K. and Balis, M.E., _Biochim. Biophys. Acta_, 474, 425 (1977).

13. Edgar, D.H. and Hope, D.B., _J. Neurochem._, 27, 949 (1976).

14. Tyce, G.M., _Res. Commun. Chem. Pathol. Pharmacol._, 16, 669 (1977).

15. Li, C.H. and Chung, D., _Nature_, 260, 622 (1976).

16. Kim, S., Galletti, P. and Paik, W.K., this volume.

17. Springer, W.R. and Koshland, D.E., Jr., _Proc. Natl. Acad. Sci. USA_, 74, 533 (1977).

18. Kort, E.N., Goy, M.F., Larsen, S.H. and Adler, J. _Proc. Natl. Acad. Sci. USA_, 72, 3939 (1975).

19. O'Dea, R.F., Viveros, O.H., Axelrod, J., Aswanikumar, S., Schiffmann, E. and Coccoran, B.A., _Nature_, 272, 462 (1978).

20. Kerr, S.J. and Borek, E., in _The Enzymes_, Boyer, P.D., Ed., Academic Press, New York, 9, 167 (1973).

21. Kerr, S.J., _Adv. Enz. Regul._, 13, 379 (1974).

14          V. Zappia *et al.*

22.   Nau, F., <u>Biochimie</u>, 58, 629  (1976).

23.   Salvatore, F. and Cimino, F., in <u>The Biochemistry of Adenosylmethionine</u>,
      Salvatore, F., Borek, E., Zappia, V., Williams-Ashman, H.G. and Schlenk, F.
      Eds., Columbia University Press, New York, 187  (1977).

24.   Cimino, F., Traboni, C., Izzo, P., and Salvatore F., in <u>Macromolecules in the</u>
      <u>Functioning Cell</u>, Salvatore, F., Marino, G., and Volpe, P. Eds., Plenum Publ.
      Co., New York, (1979) in press.

25.   Nathaus, D. and Smith, H.O., <u>Ann. Rev. Biochem.</u>, 44, 273  (1975).

26.   Sinsheimer, R.L., <u>Ann. Rev. Biochem.</u>, 46, 415  (1977).

27.   Meselson, M., Yuan, R. and Heywood, J., <u>Ann. Rev. Biochem.</u>, 41, 447  (1972).

28.   Boyer, H.W., <u>Fed. Proc.</u>, 33, 1125 (1074).

29.   Engel, J.D. and von Hippel, P.H., <u>J. Biol. Chem.</u>, 253, 927 (1978).

30.   Gannt, R., Smith, G.H. and Julian, B., <u>Virology</u>, 52, 584 (1973).

31.   Pierré, A., Berneman, A., Vedel, M., Robert-Géro, M. and Vigier, P., <u>Biochem.</u>
      <u>Biophys. Res. Commun.</u>, 81, 315  (1978).

32.   Berneman, A., Robert-Géro, N. and Vigier, P., <u>FEBS Letters</u>, 89, 33  (1978).

33.   Zappia, V., Cartení-Farina, M. and Galletti, P., in <u>The Biochemistry of Adeno-</u>
      <u>sylmethionine</u>, Salvatore, F., Borek, E., Zappia, V., Williams-Ashman, H.G. and
      Schlenk, F., Eds., Columbia University Press, New York, 473  (1977).

34.   Tabor, C.W. and Tabor, H., <u>Ann. Rev. Biochem.</u>, 45, 285  (1976).

35.   De Rosa, M., De Rosa, S., Gambacorta, A., Cartení-Farina, M. and Zappia, V.,
      <u>Biochem. Biophys. Res. Commun.</u>, 69, 253  (1976).

36.   De Rosa, M., De Rosa, S., Gambacorta, A., Cartení-Farina, M. and Zappia, V.,
      <u>Biochem. J.</u>, 174, (1978)  in press.

37.   Zappia, V., Porta, R., Cartení-Farina, M., De Rosa, M. and Gambacorta, A.,
      <u>FEBS Letters</u>, (1978) in press.

38.   Zappia, V., Galletti, P., Oliva, A., De Santis, A., <u>Anal. Biochem.</u>, 79, 535
      (1977).

39.   Lombardini, J.B., and Talalay, P., <u>Adv. Enz. Regul.</u>, 9, 349  (1971).

40.   Pietropaolo, C., Shapiro, S.K. and Salvatore, F., <u>Proc. 8th FEBS Meet.</u> Amster-
      dam, Abstr. 1044, North-Holland (1972).

41.   Gross, H.J. and Wildenauer, D., <u>Biochem. Biophys. Res. Commun.</u>, 48, 58 (1972).

42.   Swiatek, K.R., Simon, L.N. and Chao, K.L., <u>Biochemistry</u>, 12, 4670  (1973).

43.   Nishimura, S., Taya, Y., Kuchino, Y. and Ohashi, Z., <u>Biochem. Biophys. Res.</u>
      <u>Comm.</u>, 57, 702  (1974).

44.   Nishimura, S., in <u>The Biochemistry of Adenosylmethionine</u>, Salvatore, F., Borek,
      E., Zappia, V., Williams-Ashman, H.G. and Schlenk, F. Eds., Columbia University

Press, New York, 510 (1977).

45. Stoner, G.L. and Eisenberg, M.A., J. Biol. Chem., 250, 4029 (1975).

46. Stoner, G.L. and Eisenberg, M.A., J. Biol. Chem., 250, 4037 (1975).

47. Cantoni, G.L., in The Biochemistry of Adenosylmethionine, Salvatore, F., Borek, E., Zappia, V., Williams-Ashman, H.G. and Schlenk, F. Eds., Columbia University Press, New York, 557 (1977).

48. Del Re, G., Gavuzzo, E., Giglio, E., Lelj, F., Mazza, F. and Zappia, V., Acta. Cryst., B33, 3289 (1977).

49. Mudd, S.H. and Mann, J.D., J. Biol. Chem., 238, 2164 (1963).

50. Knappe, J. and Schmitt, T., Biochem. Biophys. Res. Commun., 71, 1110 (1976).

51. Zappia, V., Ayala, F., Biochim. Biophys. Acta, 268, 573 (1972).

52. Plantavid, M., Maget-Dana, R. and Douste-Blazy, L., FEBS Letters, 72, 169 (1976).

53. Stavrianapoulos, J.G. and Chargaff, E., Proc. Nat. Acad. Sci. USA, 70, 1959 (1973).

54. Stavrianapoulos, J.G., Gambino-Giuffrida, A. and Chargaff, E., Proc. Nat. Acad. Sci. USA, 73, 1087 (1976).

55. Turner, A.J., Pearson, A.G.M., Mason, R.J., this volume.

56. Duerre, J.A. and Walker, R.D., in The Biochemistry of Adenosylmethionine, Salvatore, F., Borek, E., Zappia, V., Williams-Ashman, H.G. and Schlenk, F. Eds., Columbia University Press, New York, 43 (1977).

57. Chiang, P.K., Richards, H.H. and Cantoni, G.L., Mol. Pharmacol., 13, 939 (1977).

58. Cortese, R., Perfetto, E., Arcari, P., Prota, G. and Salvatore, F., Int. J. Biochem., 5, 535 (1974).

59. Cacciapuoti, G., Oliva, A. and Zappia, V., Int. J. Biochem., 9, 35 (1978).

60. Zappia, V., Oliva, A., Cacciapuoti, G., Galletti, P., Mignucci, G. and Cartenì-Farina, M., Biochem. J., 177 (1978) in press.

61. Spence, K.D., J. Bacteriol., 106, 325 (1971).

62. Schwencke, J. and De Robichon-Szulmajster, H., Eur. J. Biochem., 65, 49 (1976).

63. Schlenk, F., in Transmethylation and Methionine Biosynthesis, Shapiro, S.K. and Schlenk, E. Eds., Univ. of Chicago Press, Chicago, 48 (1965).

64. Mizogichi, M., Parsa, I., Marsh, W.H. and Fitzgerald, P.J., Am. J. Pathol. 69, 309 (1972).

65. Stramentinoli, G., Pezzoli, C. and Galli-Kienle, M., Biochem. Pharmacol., (1978) in press.

66. Zappia, V., Galletti, P., Porcelli, M., Ruggiero, G., Andreana, A., FEBS Let-

<u>ters</u>, 90, 331 (1978).

67. Pezzoli, C., Stramentinoli, G. and Galli-Kienle, M., <u>Biochem. Biophys. Res. Commun.</u>, (1978) in press.

68. Smith, J.D., <u>Biochem. Biophys. Res. Commun.</u>, 73, 7 (1976).

# The Chemical Properties of Sulfonium Compounds

## Alberto Fiecchi

Istituto di Chimica della Facoltà di Medicina e Chirurgia
Università di Milano, via Saldini, 50 20133 Milano, Italia

The interest in natural sulfonium compounds is linked to the unique role of these substances in enzymatic reactions implying a group transfer. The present paper deals with some recent advances in knowledge of the chemical properties of the three most important members of this series, S-methylmethionine, (SMM), S-adenosyl-methionine, (SAM), and its decarboxylated derivative, S-adenosyl-5'-methylthiopropylamine, (deca SAM).

## REACTIONS OF S-METHYLMETHIONINE

SMM, also called vitamin U, occurs in a variety of higher plants. Its salts are implicated in shay ulcers of rats. The crystal structure of SMM chloride hydrochloride has been very recently determined by Del Re, et al. (1). The sulfonium group is pyramidal, with the carbon-sulfur bonds and the angles around the sulfur atom nearly equal (Fig. 1).

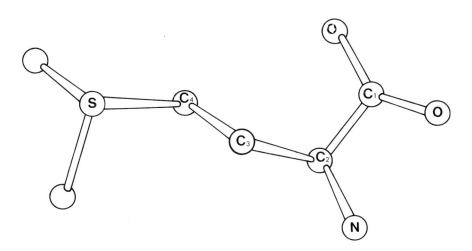

Fig. 1. Crystal structure of SMM

The behavior of SMM salts in aqueous solutions has been recently reexamined by
Ramirez et al. (2).   In basic and neutral solutions the main decomposition pathway
leads to homoserine and dimethyl sulfide via homoserine lactone (Fig. 2).   The evaluation of the half-life (t1/2) of SMM at 90°and at various pH values shows that
the decomposition rate is maximal at basic pH's and decreases markedly when the pH
is decreased.   These facts are in agreement with the calculations of Del Re, et al.
(1), who showed that the cyclic conformations, with the carboxyl group near the
sulfur atom, are strongly stabilized.   It can be concluded that serine lactone is
probably formed by an intramolecular group participation of the carboxyl group.

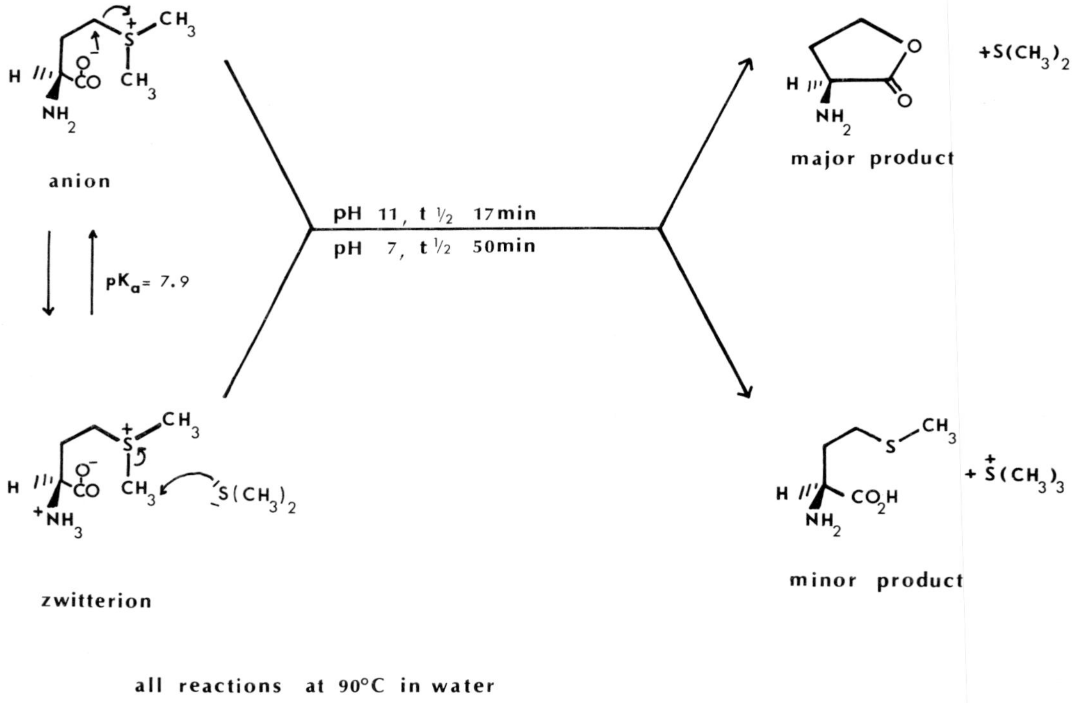

all reactions at 90°C in water

Fig. 2.   Reactions of SMM at basic and neutral pH's.

A second pathway of SMM decomposition has been detected, i.e., a nucleophilic attack of dimethyl sulfide on the methyl group of SMM; this pathway leads to methionine.   The specific rate of this reaction appears to be relatively small, probably
due to the low solubility of dimethyl sulfide in water.   The reaction, however,
plays an important role at acidic pH's.   Minute amounts of homocysteine are also
formed, probably by a very slow nucleophilic attack of dimethyl sulfide on methionine (Fig. 3).

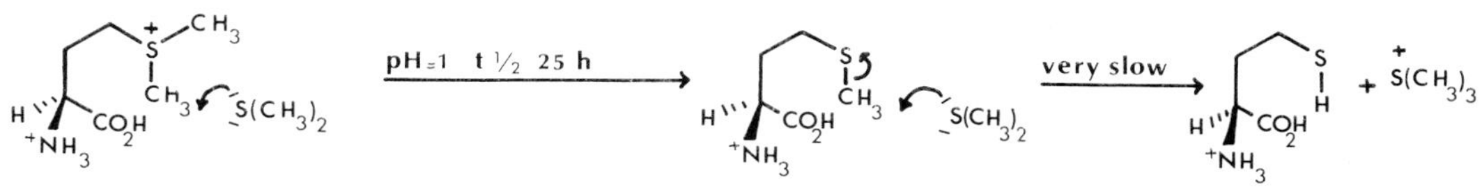

Fig. 3.   Reactions of SMM at acidic pH.

## REACTIONS OF S-ADENOSYLMETHIONINE

SAM was discovered by Cantoni, who, on the basis of biochemical evidence, proposed
a structure (3), which was later confirmed by degradation and synthesis.  For a
long time SAM was used only for biochemical studies, owing to the thermal instability of its salts.  It was recently discovered that SAM forms a number of salts
which are stable enough to allow pharmacological experimentation and use (4).  General formulas of these compounds are: SAM.3RSO$_3$H; SAM.2H$_2$SO$_4$.RSO$_3$H; SAM respectively,
with R= -CH$_3$-C$_2$H$_5$, -4-CH$_3$C$_6$H$_5$, etc.

The behavior of SAM is much more complex, when compared to that of SMM.  Most of the
tested reactions give rise to complex mixtures and only the principal components have
been identified.  A few reactions, which have been recently reexamined, will be considered here.  At slightly acidic pH's, SAM reacts in a way similar to SMM, giving
rise to methylthioadenosine in addition to homoserine (5).  The participation of the
carboxyl group in the cleavage of the carbon-sulfur bond between the sulfur atom
and the amino acid residue has been hypothesized (1,3).

Differences in the behavior of SAM and SMM are shown at pH 12 (Fig. 4).  At this
pH, the N-glycosidic bond of SAM is cleaved at room temperature and formation of
adenine is observed in addition to a compound which has been considered to be a
pentosylmethionine (6).  Cornforth et al. have recently demonstrated that treatment
of the pentosylmethionine with periodate ions gives rise to S-carboxylmethylmethio-
nine instead of the expected S-carbonylmethylmethionine (7).  As a consequence, the
authors hypothesized that hydroxide ions transform the intermediary vinylsulfo-
nium compound into a β-dicarbonyl derivative, which would give the acid by treatment with periodate ions.  S-carboxymethylmethionine was used by the authors for
the evaluation of the absolute configuration of the sulfur atom.  For this purpose,
the two isomers (A and B) of the acid were synthesized and separated by ion-exchange
chromatography.  The "Rectus" absolute configuration of the sulfur atom in the i-
somer B was determined by X-ray diffraction and this isomer was shown to be different from the isomer A, obtained from natural SAM.  It was deduced that natural SAM

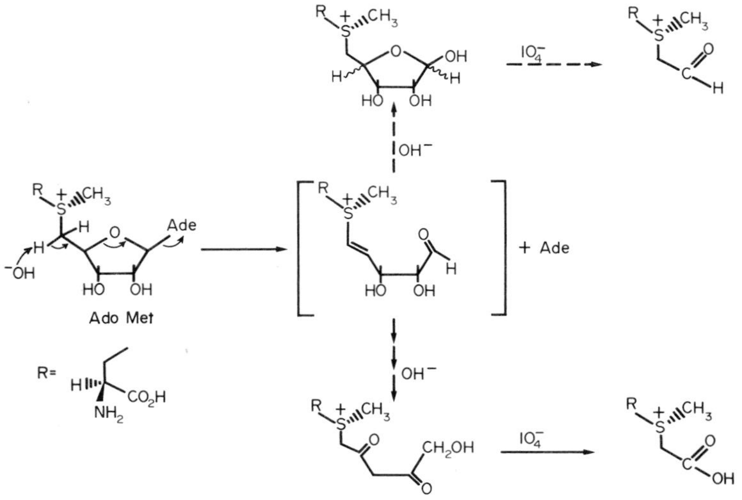

Fig. 4.   Hypothesized formation of S-carboxymethylmethionine from SAM

has the "Sinister" configuration at sulfur atom.  Chemical demethylation of SAM
occurs with fairly good yields by treatment of SAM with iodide ions at 50° for 24
hours (8), to yield S-adenosylhomocysteine (SAH) (Fig. 5).

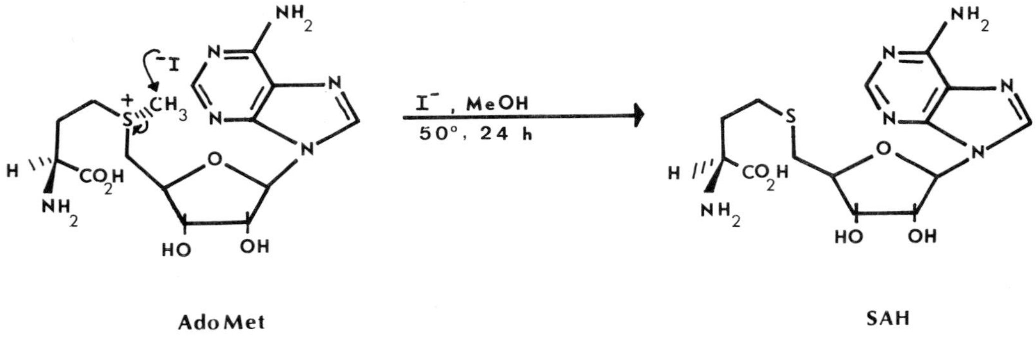

**AdoMet**                                                                **SAH**

Fig. 5.   Reaction of SAM with iodide ions.

Quantitative decarboxylation of SAM was demonstrated by Zappia et al. to occur in
the presence of pyridoxal-5'-phosphate (PLP) and copper ions (9,10).  The intermediary formation of a Schiff base was demonstrated on the basis of the optimal pH
value for the reaction.  The formation of a chelate with the copper ions may explain
the catalytic action of the metal (Fig. 6).  It is worth noting that the sulfonium

ion seems to stabilize the Schiff base and to be essential for decarboxylation. In fact, slow formation of the Schiff base and no decarboxylation were observed when such natural sulfides as SAH and methionine were treated with PLP and copper ions. The formation of a Schiff base from SAM was recently confirmed on the basis of UV spectral data (11,12).

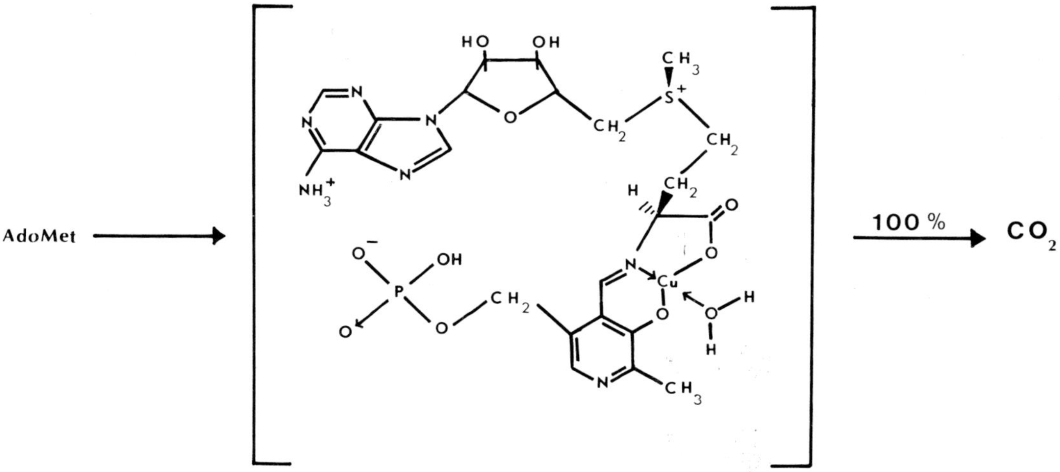

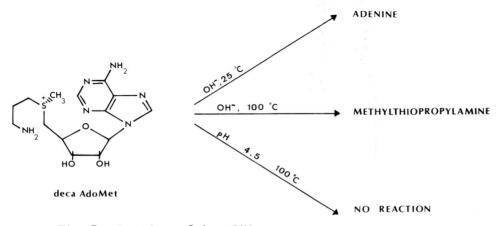

Fig. 6.  Possible structure of the chelate of the Schiff base formed from SAM and PLP.

REACTIONS OF S-ADENOSYL-5'-METHYLTHIOPROPYLAMINE

Despite the key intermediary role of decarboxylated SAM (deca SAM) in polyamine biosynthesis, a fairly small number of biochemical and chemical studies have been performed with this compound due to poor availaibility.  The chemical behavior of deca SAM was studied by Zappia et al. (13), (Fig. 7).

Fig. 7.  Reactions of deca SAM

At room temperature and at basic pH, adenine is formed from deca SAM by cleavage of the glycosidic bond, as in the case of SAM, on raising the temperature to 100°C, further degradation occurs.   These degradation procedures were utilized to confirm the structure of synthetic sulfonium nucleosides (14).   No degradation of the molecule is observed at the acidic pH which causes the cleavage of the carbon–sulfur bond of SAM.   This result further indicates the intervention of the carboxyl group in the cleavage of the carbon–sulfur bond.   Recently a method was developed by Zappia et al. for the separation of deca SAM from SAM, based on the recovery of deca SAM after degradation of SAM at acidic pH (15).   By this method, pure deca SAM was obtained by these authors after enzymatic decarboxylation of SAM.

It appears from the data shown that little is known about the chemical behavior of natural sulfonium compounds.   This seems mainly due to difficulties in the analysis of the complex reaction mixtures.   High performance liquid chromatography (HPLC) appears to be very promising for the solution of this problem.   It was first shown by Hoffman that SAM is well separated by HPLC from its demethylated analog, SAH (16).   The author describes a method for the chromatographic measurement of these nucleosides in 1 g of tissue or less, using a cation exchanger and eluting formate gradient.

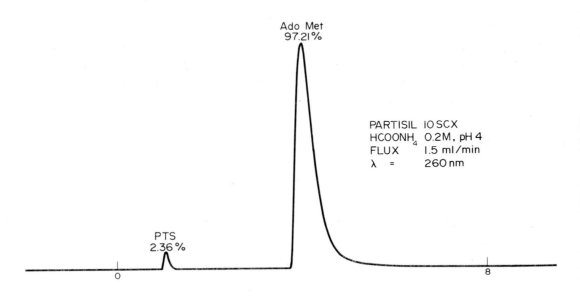

Fig. 8.   HPLC trace of disulfate, p-toluenesulfonate of SAM.   (PTS, p-toluenesulfonic acid).

This method was utilized to evaluate the purity of the disulfate, the p-toluenesulfonate of SAM (Fig. 8).  It has been shown that 97.21% and 2.36% of the total UV absorbance at 260nm is associated with SAM and p-toluenesulfonic acid, respectively; the residual 0.43% is due to minute amounts of impurities.

## REFERENCES

1)  Del Re, C., Gavuzzo, E., Giglio, E., Lelj, F., Mazza, F. and Zappia, V., Acta Cryst. B 33, 3289 (1977).

2)  Ramirez, F., Finnan, J.L. and Carlson, M., J. Org. Chem. 15, 2597 (1973).

3)  Cantoni, G.L., J. Am. Chem. Soc. 74, 2942 (1952).

4)  Bioresearch, Ltd., U.S. Patents No. 3,893,999; 3,954,726; 4,028,183; 4,047,686.

5)  De La Haba, G., Jamieson, G.A., Mudd, S.H. and Richards, H.H., J. Am.Chem Soc. 81, 3975 (1959).

6)  Parks, L.W. and Schlenk, F., J. Biol. Chem. 230, 295 (1958).

7)  Cornforth, J.W., Reichard, S.A., Talalay, P., Carrell, H.L. and Glusker, J.P., J. Am. Chem. Soc. 99, 7292 (1977).

8)  Boehringer Mannheim G.M.B.H., B. R. P. Anmeldung P 1,795,282.

9)  Zappia, V., Carteni Farina, M. and Galletti, P., Abstr. Symposium on Organic Sulphur Chemistry (Lund) p. II A23 (1972).

10) Zappia, V., Carteni Farina, M. and Galletti, P., in The Biochemistry of Adenosyl-methionine, Salvatore, F., Borek, E., Zappia, V., Williams Ashman, H.G. and Schlenk, F., Eds., Columbia University Press, New York, 473 (1977).

11) Trewyn, R.W., Nakamura, K.D., O'Connor, M.L. and Parks, L.W., Biochim. Biophys. Acta 327, 336 (1973).

12) Borchardt, R.T., Wu, Y.S. and Wu, B.S., Biochem. Pharmac. 27, 120 (1978).

13) Zappia, V., Zyder-Cwick, C.R. and Schlenk, F., J. Biol. Chem. 244, 4499 (1969).

14) Borchardt, R.T., Wu, Y.S., Huber, J.A. and Wycpalek, A.F., J. Med. Chem. 19, 1104 (1976).

15) Zappia, V., Galletti, P., Oliva, A. and De Santis, A., Anal. Biochem. 79, 535 (1977).

16) Hoffman, J., Anal. Biochem. 68, 522 (1975).

# Analysis and Distribution of Adenosylmethionine and Adenosylhomocysteine in Mammalian Tissues

**Terho O. Eloranta**

Department of Biochemistry, University of Kuopio, POB 138, SF-70101, Kuopio 10, Finland

Since the discovery of adenosylmethionine (SAM) by Cantoni in the early fifties, the enzyme machinery responsible for the formation and catabolism of this compound has been rather well characterized in a variety of biological sources (for references, see 1,2). Some knowledge has also been accumulated about the levels of SAM and their pharmacological control in certain mammalian tissues (2-4). However, only a few extensive studies have been published on the distribution of SAM in animal tissues (5,6), and the factors affecting its tissue concentrations are still poorly known.

## FORMATION AND REGULATORY CONSEQUENCES OF ADENOSYLHOMOCYSTEINE IN THE METABOLISM OF ADENOSYLMETHIONINE

SAM links together two physiologically important processes: biological methylation and polyamine biosynthesis (Fig. 1). Evidently a great majority of SAM is utilized in a number of methylation reactions (7) producing nucleic acids and proteins of modified stability, activity and function, less toxic products, physiologically important low molecular-weight compounds and, in addition, adenosylhomocysteine (SAH), which is known to be a potent inhibitor of most of these reactions (1,2,8). Under normal conditions SAH can be rapidly degraded to homocysteine and adenosine by a specific hydrolase (2,8). Homocysteine is further catabolized via the transsulfuration pathway (7) and adenosine is effectively degraded to ribose 1-phosphate and uric acid or allantoin in the animals possessing urate oxidase activity (9,10). Although the transsulfuration pathway does not appear to be operative in rat lung, heart and testes (7) or in ruminant heart and skeletal muscle (11), probably all mammalian tissues contain at least one enzyme capable of metabolizing homocysteine (7). However, any condition leading to the accumulation of either homocysteine or, especially, adenosine might be expected to block the catabolism of SAH, since the hydrolase reaction greatly favors the synthetic direction (8). Accumulation of SAH would then be expected to inhibit the catabolism of SAM. Since the rate of SAM formation seems to be controlled by tissue methionine concentration (2,6),

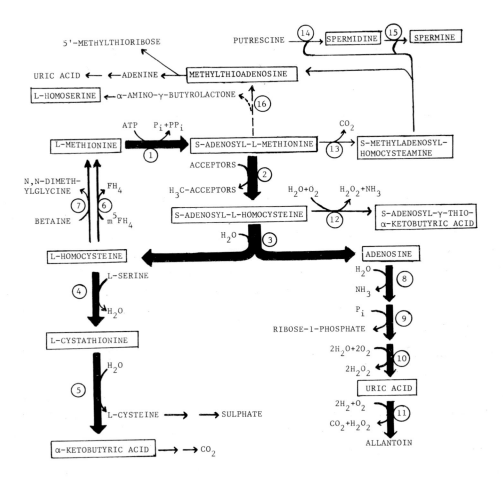

Fig. 1.  Metabolism of SAM in animal tissues. Numbers indicate the following enzymes: 1 = methionine adenosyltransferase, 2 = methyltransferases, 3 = S-adenosylhomocysteine hydrolase, 4 = cysta-
thionine β-synthase, 5 = cystathionase, 6 = $m^5FH_4$: homocysteine
methyltransferase, 7 = betaine: homocysteine methyltransferase,
8 = adenosine deaminase, 9 = inosine-guanosine phosphorylase,
10 = xanthine oxidase, 11 = urate oxidase, 12 = amino acid
oxidase, 13 = S-adenosyl-L-methionine decarbcxylase, 14 =
spermidine synthase, 15 = spermine synthase, 16 = SAM splitting
enzyme.

its production might proceed independently of the rate of its catabolism.  Cata-
bolic routes of SAM (12,13) and SAH (9) other than the transsulfuration pathway
reported to operate in some tissues, are unlikely to play any controlling role due
to their limited capacity (13) and distribution (9,12).  Thus, the concentration of

SAH might be expected to regulate not only the important metabolic functions of SAM but also its tissue concentrations. Therefore, the simultaneous analysis of both SAM and SAH is desirable to unravel the possible interrelationships between the physiological functions and tissue concentrations of SAM.

QUANTITATION OF ADENOSYLMETHIONINE AND ADENOSYLHOMOCYSTEINE FROM TISSUES

The methods used for the quantitative analysis of SAM can be classified into two types: the first based on the use of a specific methyl transfer reaction (4,14,15) and the other on the use of ion exchange resins (5,10,16-19). Some of the methods still commonly in use are compared with each other in Table 1. Due to their high

TABLE I.   COMPARISON OF SOME METHODS USED FOR THE QUANTITATION OF S-ADENOSYLMETH-
IONINE (SAM) AND S-ADENOSYLHOMOCYSTEINE (SAH) FROM TISSUE SAMPLES

| Principle | Sensi-tivity (nmoles) | Approx. time consumption/one person | | Reference |
| --- | --- | --- | --- | --- |
| | | h/sample | h/30 samples | |
| Enzymic-isotopic methods for the analysis of SAM only | | | | |
| Measurement of the radioactivity ratio $^3H/^{14}C$ of ($^{14}CH_3$: $^3H$)melatonin formed from endogenous and $^{14}CH_3$-labelled SAM in the presence of excess amounts of N-($^3H$)acetylserotonin and hydroxyindole O-methyl transferase | 2 | 4 | 6 | (14,15) |
| Measurement of the formation of ($^3H$) methylhistamine from endogenous and $^3H$-labelled SAM in the presence of excess amounts of histamine and histamine methyl transferase | 0.1 | 4 | 6 | (4) |
| Chromatographic methods for the analysis of both SAM and SAH | | | | |
| Separation of SAM by Dowex 50-Na$^+$ and SAH by Dowex 50-H$^+$; precipitation, alkaline hydrolysis and Dowex 50-H$^+$; estimation of UV-absorbance | 300 (for SAM) 500 (for SAH) | 4 8 | 12 60 | (5) (18) |
| Separation of SAM and SAH by high-pressure liquid chromatography; estimation of UV-absorbance | 50 | 2.5 | 45 | (19) |
| Separation of SAM and SAH by Cellex-H$^+$; estimation of UV-absorbance | 100 | 6 | 16 | |

sensitivity and absolute specificity, the enzymic-isotopic methods can be prefered
to the chromatographic ones whenever only small amounts of tissue are available for
SAM detection.  However, only chromatographic techniques have been developed for
the simultaneous analysis of SAM and SAH.  Since both of these compounds are strong
cations their complete separation from each other and from a variety of other u.v.-
absorbing cations present in acid tissue extracts has turned out to be difficult
when strong cation exchangers are used.  The first chromatographic method ensuring
reliable quantitation of SAM and SAH from tissue samples was based on the separation
and purification of these compounds by several successive column chromatographies
and estimation of the ribose moiety by the orcinol reaction (17).  The great time
consumption, which was a serious drawback of this method, has been significantly
reduced in the improved column chromatographic (5,19) and high-pressure liquid
chromatographic (HPLC) methods (18) now available.  Of the modern HPLC methods, that
published by Schatz et al. (10) is about 10 times as sensitive and rapid as that
developed by Hoffman (18), but it has not yet been modified for the detection of
SAM.  Thus, even the improved methods suitable for simultaneous analysis of SAM and
SAH are still rather insensitive, requiring gram-amounts of tissue samples, and
are too time-consuming to be considered for use in routine analysis.  By appropriate
decreases in the column size and in the elution volumes, the sensitivity of the
simple column chromatographic method developed by our group (19) compares favorably
with that reported by Hoffman (18).  Since free ribose or ribose-containing u.v.-
absorbing contaminants are unlikely to be present in SAH or SAM fractions, the use
of the orcinol reaction instead of u.v.-absorptivity might further confirm the
specificity of the method.  Nevertheless, it is useful as such, for SAM and SAH
determinations from most tissues (the spleen and kidneys appear to be exceptions),
and is cheap and simple.  It takes advantage of the charge difference between SAM,
SAH, other nucleoside derivatives and u.v.-absorbing bases at slightly acidic pH
and the weak binding ability of a phosphocellulose cation exchanger, Cellex-P.  As
shown in Fig. 2, most of the contaminating u.v.-absorbing material present in ether-
extracted trichloroacetic acid supernatants of tissue homogenates is bound only
loosely or not at all to Cellex-P ($H^+$ form) and is easily eluted with 1mM-HCl.  To
elute adenine (and probably other free bases), 10 mM-HCl is required.  After that,
only SAH and SAM are retained and can easily be separated by a stepwise HCl-gradeint.
The quantitation of both substances is achieved by measuring $E_{257}$ of the corresponding fractions, using a molar extinction coefficient of 15,000 liter·$mol^{-1}$ $cm^{-1}$ and
correcting the results by the recovery of the radioactive internal standards added
to the tissue samples before homogenization with trichloroacetic acid.  Trichloroacetic acid is preferred to perchloric acid since it can be removed by ether extraction.  Removal of extra perchloric acid involves addition of cations, which can
hamper the binding of SAH and SAM to the resin.  Due to the limited binding capacity

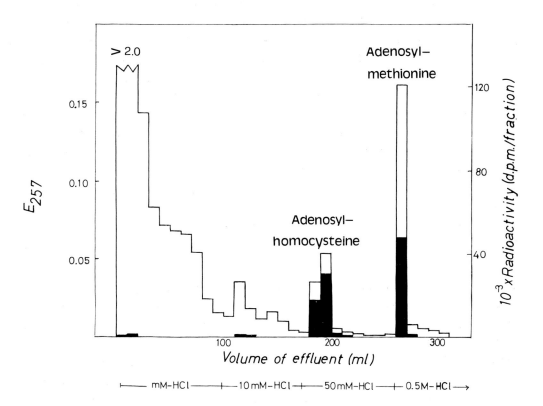

Fig. 2. Separation of SAH and SAM from liver extract by phosphocellulose
column chromatography. A 12 ml sample of rat liver homogenate
was added with S-adenosyl-L-[Me-$^{14}$C]methionine (82500 d.p.m.)
and S-[8-$^{14}$C]adenosyl-L-homocysteine (87750 d.p.m.) and immediately mixed with 2.5 ml of ice-cold 50% (w/v) trichloroacetic
acid. After centrifugation, the supernatant was extracted three
times with ether. A 9.0 ml portion of the supernatant, corresponding to 1.86 g of wet liver, was applied to a Cellex-P (H$^{+}$
form) column (1 cm x 7 cm). The column was eluted with a stepwise HCl gradient by collecting 10 ml fractions as shown in the
Figure. Absorbance was read at 257 nm, and radioactivities of
samples of the effluent were counted. Radioactivity is shown
by black and E$_{257}$ by white columns. About 87% of radioactive
SAH present in the tissue extract was recovered in the first 20
ml of 50 mM-HCl effluent and 93% of radioactive SAM in the first
10 ml of 0.5 M-HCl effluent. Adenosine, hypoxanthine and inosine were eluted with 1 mM HCl. To elute adenine from the column 10 mM HCl was required. Reproduced from (19), with the
permission of the Biochemical Society.

of Cellex-P, any overloading by cations should be avoided. Endogenous cations
present in tissue extracts do not present any difficulties provided that the ratio
(1 g of tissue)/(2 cm$^3$ of resin bed) is not exceeded. When used for preparative
purposes, the presence of buffer cations in the acid solution may cause troubles.
This is especially true for the preparation of SAM, whose enzymic synthesis involves very high Mg$^{2+}$ and K$^+$ concentrations; a significant dilution of the incubation mixture before chromatography is required to avoid losses of SAM. However,
the method is very suitable for the purification of SAM preparations and for the
preparation of SAH. Since SAH, unlike SAM, is fairly acid-labile, the use of a
weaker acid instead of HCl is recommended in preparative chromatography. All the
impurities released by 1 and 10 mM-HCl, including, e.g., adenosine and adenine and
their degradation products, can also be eluted with 1 M formic acid. Thereafter,
pure SAH can be collected with 10 M formic acid, evaporated to dryness at 20-30°C
without any hydrolysis to adenine, re-dissolved in water and stored frozen. Due to
its high u.v. absorbance and inability to release SAM from the phosphocellulose
column, formic acid is less suitable for analytical chromatography.

Although the improved separation and quantitation techniques for SAM and SAH from
tissue extracts appear to be rather specific, the rapid degradation of these compounds might cause misleading results for their tissue concentrations. Destruction
during separation processes is easily corrected for by the aid of radioactive internal standards, but any degradation occurring between the killing of the animal
and treatment of the removed organs or tissues with acid is not controllable. I
studied the stability of endogenous SAM and SAH in rat liver preparations in greater
detail and noticed that SAM was effectively converted to SAH both in whole tissues
and especially in tissue homogenates prepared in sucrose solution even at temper-
atures close to zero (6). This degradation may be connected with the high SAM-degrading activity present in the soluble cytosol fraction of liver homogenates.
This activity which is entirely dependent on dialysable low-molecular weight compounds, can be restored by the addition of glycine to dialyzed enzyme preparation
and appears to produce SAH, which is rapidly catabolized further (Eloranta, T.O.,
unpublished results). All these observations suggest an important role for so-
called competing methyltransferases in the catabolism of SAM. Even the SAM de-
carboxylating activity, dependent on membrane-bound enzymes (20), is probably just
an extension of the demethylation-transsulfuration route leading to the conversion
of SAM to α-ketobutyrate, which is then degraded to propionyl-CoA and CO$_2$ by membrane-bound enzyme machinery (Eloranta, T.O. and Raina, A.M., unpublished results).

The SAM-degrading activity of the cytosol fraction is not limited to liver only,
but appears to be present in all the tissues we have examined. In fact, the activ-

ity per g wet weight of tissue is highest in the kidneys and close to that of liver in the uterus, lungs, prostate and small intestine, whereas it appears to be rather low in brain, pancreas, thymus, spleen, heart and skeletal muscle. These results are in good accord with the apparent turn-over rate of SAM, reported to be much more rapid in the liver ($t_{1/2}$ ~ 10 min) than in the brain and spleen (2,3). Anyway, to get a reliable view of the tissue distribution of SAM and SAH, the tissues should be rapidly frozen, preferably in situ, and not allowed to melt before homogenization in acid, whenever an immediate acid treatment after killing is not possible.

## TISSUE DISTRIBUTION OF ADENOSYLMETHIONINE AND ADENOSYLHOMOCYSTEINE

Although the concentration range of SAM and SAH has been known for several mammalian tissues for many years, the first systematic exploration of their distribution has been reported only recently in rat tissues (6). In general, the SAM concentrations shown in Table 2 agree well with those reported by Salvatore et al. (5), but are

TABLE 2.  DISTRIBUTION OF ADENOSYLMETHIONINE, ADENOSYLHOMOCYSTEINE, METHIONINE AD-ENOSYLTRANSFERASE AND ADENOSYLHOMOCYSTEINE HYDROLASE IN RAT TISSUES[a]

| Tissue | S-Adenosylmethionine (nmol/g of wet tissue) | | S-Adenosyl-homocysteine (nmol/g wet tissue) | Methionine adenosyl-transferase (pmol/min per mg of protein) | S-Adenosyl-homocysteine hydrolase (nmol/min per mg of protein) |
|---|---|---|---|---|---|
| Adrenals | (25) | 51.5 | 16.1 | 86 | 11.7 |
| Brain | (4) | 25.4±0.9 | 3.4±1.2 | 43±10 | 11.6±1.5 |
| Epididymal fat | (6) | <4.0 | <2.0 | 22 | 7.7 |
| Heart | (17) | 38.5 | 3.9 | 42 | 6.3 |
| Kidneys | (8) | 47.2* | 22.5±3.4 | 192±36 | 25.0±0.0 |
| Liver | (2) | 67.5±1.1 | 43.8±3.2 | 7700±160 | 51.1±6.5 |
| Lungs | (4) | 31.2±1.3 | 3.7±0.3 | 38±11 | 5.9±1.1 |
| Pancreas | (20) | 39.8 | 11.4 | 558 | 59.9 |
| Skeletal muscle | (4) | 22.7±2.1 | 4.7±0.7 | 13 | 9.4 |
| Small intestine | (4) | 32.6 | 3.7 | 83 | 10.5 |
| Spleen | (14) | 42.2* | 6.4* | 65 | 10.0 |
| Testes | (11) | 21.3 | 5.9 | 70±6 | 7.0±0.9 |
| Ventral Prostate | (25) | 59.5 | 10.4 | 141 | 4.7 |

[a]Male rats aged 6 weeks and fed ad libitum were used for analysis. The values represent one pooled preparation or the mean (±S.D.) of three pooled preparations, each obtained from the number of organs indicated in parentheses. *Determined after electrophoretic purification. Reproduced from (6), with the permission of the Biochemical Society.

somewhat lower than those reported earlier (2), which is partly due to differences in molar extinction coefficients used for calculations (3) but may also indicate higher specificity of the present methods. Even the specificity of the phosphocellulose column-chromatographic method turned out to be unsatisfactory for the kidneys, which appeared to contain about equal amounts of SAM and a u.v.-absorbing compound able to bind to Cellex as tightly as SAM. The contaminant was easily separated from SAM by paper electrophoresis at pH 4.3. Since it appeared to be as cationic as SAM but migrated more slowly towards the cathode in the electric field, a molecular size significantly greater than that of SAM can be assumed.

SAH concentrations have been previously reported only for a few rat tissues (5), and the values measured significantly exceed the present ones.

On the basis of the distribution pattern shown in Table 2, the following conclusions may be drawn:

   a) The concentration of SAM exceeds that of SAH in all rat tissues.

   b) Except for fat, in which only trace amounts of SAM and SAH can be detected, differences in the concentration of SAM between different tissues are not dramatic and reveal no correlation with the great variation in the distribution of the activity of methionine adenosyltransferase.

   c) All tissues appear to be provided with a significantly higher capacity to catabolize SAH than to synthesize SAM.

Since very little is known about the distribution of SAM and SAH in other animals, these conclusions might be valid only for the rat. However, at least in mouse brain (4,21), in the liver of mouse (18), rabbit and calf (5), and in the kidney, lung, brain and skeletal muscle of rabbit (5) the concentrations of SAM and SAH are very close to the values for the corresponding rat tissues. Thus, distribution studies in the rat might provide information which may be also generally applicable to other mammals.

In general, tissue SAM concentrations appear to be close to saturating as to the function of, e.g., mammalian protein and nucleic acid transmethylases, reported to have $K_M$-values of 1-5 $\mu$M for SAM, but are clearly lower than the 100-180 $\mu$M $K_M$-values calculated for "competing" systems, e.g. glycine N-methyltransferase (22,23). On the other hand, SAH concentrations in all tissues, except fat, appear to exceed the 0.1-2.1 $\mu$M $K_i$-values of, e.g., DNA and histone methylases (24), tRNA methyltransferases (23), phenylethanolamine N-methyltransferase and acetylserotonin O-methyltransferase (25), but are lower than that measured for glycine N-methyltransferase (23). All this is appropriate for maintaining tissue SAM concentrations at a fairly constant level, but as to the important metabolic functions of SAM, the SAH concentrations seem to be unfavorably high in many tissues. For example, according to the results obtained in vitro, the hepatic SAH concentrations should be expected to entirely block most of the methylation reactions involved in the synthesis of some physiologically important compounds and in the stabilization and functional modification of nucleic acids and proteins. This disproportion may indicate that even the present values for tissue SAH concentrations are overestimates due either to methodological unspecificity or to the rapid conversion of SAM to SAH during tissue preparation. However, it should be kept in mind that we do not have any experimental knowledge of the possible compartmentalization of these compounds in mammalian cells. It should also be noted that there is some experimental evidence of the ability of SAH to pass through the cell membranes from the inside to the outside, although the reverse process does not seem to occur (8,26), which indicates that part of the SAH present in tissues might be extracellular. If this is the case, significant concentrations of SAH could be expected to be found in blood and urine. However, the accuracy of these speculations remains to be established.

## FLUCTUATIONS OF THE TISSUE CONCENTRATIONS OF ADENOSYLMETHIONINE AND ADENOSYLHOMO-CYSTEINE

To clarify the fluctuation ranges for SAM and SAH in tissues, we studied the effects of a variety of conditions on their concentrations, mainly in the liver. Treatment with cortisol did not appear to change the concentration of hepatic SAM and only slightly increased that of SAH, although it resulted in a significant stimulation of the enzyme activities responsible for the synthesis of SAM and degradation of SAH (27). Since the tissue distribution of these compounds was similar in both sexes (6), it seems reasonable to assume that neither sex steroids play any central role in the control of their tissue concentrations. Also the hormonal changes during developmental growth did not appear to alter hepatic SAM concentration, whereas SAH concentration was clearly increased during the period of rapid growth (6). During regenerative growth of the liver, after partial hepatectomy or treatment with thioacetamide, no change was noticed in the hepatic concentration of either compound (27). The significantly lower SAH concentration in the liver of new-born rats as compared to that of young adults (6) is somewhat unexpected, since the transsulfuration pathway (involved in the catabolism of SAH) seems to become more active with age (28). However, the explanation might be found from nutritional differences affecting tissue methionine supply and the activity of the homocysteine remethylation cycle. In the brain, the concentration of SAM appeared to decrease slightly with age, whereas that of SAH remained fairly unchanged (6).

Unlike growth processes and hormonal changes, methionine administration caused a dramatic increase in the hepatic concentrations of SAM and SAH (6). The effects

of the changes in the ntUritional state of the animal (27) can probably be attributed to changes in methionine supply.  However, even a two-week methionine deprivation was not able to decrease the hepatic SAM level (27), which probably em-
phasizes the effectiveness of homocysteine remethylation during limited methionine
supply.  On the other hand, the dramatic effect of methionine on SAM accumulation
could be prevented markedly by simultaneous glycine administration (6).  Since the
uptake of methionine into the liver was observed to be unaffected by glycine, it
appears that glycine stimulates the consumption of SAM.  The lack of any significant
SAH accumulation in response to stimulated SAM utilization can be explained by the
very high capacity of SAH hydrolase, adenosine catabolism and the transsulfuration
route.

We have also studied the effect of disturbed SAH catabolism on liver SAM concentration.  Since the transsulfuration pathway includes two pyridoxal-dependent enzymes
(7), a prolonged pyridoxine deprivation could be expected to block the reaction
route; that is just what seemed to happen (19).  The effect of $B_6$-deprivation on
the catabolism of SAH in the liver is clearly deleterious.  The apparent decrease
in hepatic SAH level during more prolonged $B_6$-deprivation might be due to increased
SAH excretion, although the concentration of SAH in the urine or in tissues other
than the liver was not studied.  Anyway, it seems most interesting that even under
the drastic metabolic disturbances probably created by SAH accumulation the concentration of SAM still remains unaffected.

In conclusion, it appears that the rate of SAM synthesis and accumulation in rat
tissues is controlled by the available methionine.  Al least the hepatic methionine
concentration is probably maintained fairly constant under physiological conditions
by a mechanism involving both an effective homocysteine remethylation cycle and a
SAM-consuming system rather insensitive to SAH.

## REFERENCES

1.  Salvatore, F., Borek, E., Zappia, V., Williams-Ashman, H.G. and Schlenk, F.,
    Eds., The Biochemistry of Adenosylmethionine, Columbia University Press, New
    York (1977).

2.  Lombardini, J.B. and Talalay, P., Adv. Enz. Regul. 9, 349 (1971).

3.  Baldessarini, R.J., Int. Rev. Neurobiol. 18, 41 (1975).

4.  Taylor, K.M., and Randall, P.K., J. Pharmacol. Exp. Ther. 194, 303 (1975).

5.  Salvatore, F., Utili, R., Zappia, V., and Shapiro, S.K., Anal. Biochem. 41,
    16 (1971).

6.  Eloranta, T.O., Biochem. J. 166, 521 (1977).

7.  Finkelstein, J.D., _Metab. Clin. Exp._ 23, 387 (1974).

8.  Walker, D.R. and Duerre, J.A., _Can. J. Biochem._ 53, 312 (1975).

9.  Cortese, R., Perfetto, E., Arcari, P., Prota, G. and Salvatore, F., _Int. J. Biochem._ 5, 535 (1974).

10. Schatz, R.A., Vunnam, C.R. and Sellinger, O.Z., _Life Sci._ 20, 375 (1977).

11. Radcliffe, B.C. and Egan, A.R. _Aust. J. Biol. Sci._ 27, 465 (1977).

12. Swiatek, K.R., Simon, L.N. and Chao, K.-L., _Biochemistry_ 12, 4670 (1973).

13. Pegg, A.E. and Williams-Ashman, H.G., _Biochem. J._ 115, 241 (1969).

14. Baldessarini, R.J. and Kopin, I.J., _Anal. Biochem._ 6, 289 (1963).

15. Baldessarini, R.J. and Kopin, I.J., _J. Neurochem._ 13, 769 (1966).

16. Shapiro, S.K. and Ehninger, D.J., _Anal. Biochem._ 15, 323 (1966).

17. Gaitonde, M.K. and Gaull, G.E., _Biochem. J._ 102, 959 (1967).

18. Hoffman, J., _Anal. Biochem._ 68, 522 (1975).

19. Eloranta, T.O., Kajander, E.O and Raina, A.M., _Biochem. J._ 160, 287 (1976).

20. Sturman, J.A., _Biochim. Biophys. Acta_ 428, 56 (1976).

21. Schatz, R.A., Vunnam, C.R. and Sellinger, O.Z., _Neurochem. Res._ 2, 27 (1977).

22. Barman, T.E., in _Enzyme Handbook, Supplement I_ Springer-Verlag, Berlin-Heidelberg-New York, 168 (1974).

23. Kerr, S.J., in _Control Processes in Neoplasia_, M.A. Mehlman and R.W. Hanson, Eds., Academic Press, New York, 83 (1974).

24. Duerre, J.A. and Walker, R.D., in _The Biochemistry of Adenosylmethionine_, F. Salvatore, E. Borek, V. Zappia, H.G. Williams-Ashman, and F. Schlenk, Eds. Columbia University Press, New York, 43 (1977).

25. Deguchi, T. and Barchas, J., _J. Biol. Chem._ 246, 3175 (1971).

26. Miller, C.H. and Duerre, J.A., _J. Biol. Chem._ 244, 4237 (1969).

27. Eloranta, T.O. and Raina, A.M., _Biochem. J._ 168, 179 (1977).

28. Finkelstein, J.D., _Arch. Biochem. Biophys._ 122, 583 (1967).

# Protein Methylation: Perspectives in Central Nervous System

## Sangduk Kim, Patricia Galletti and Woon Ki Paik

The Fels Research Institute, Temple University School of Medicine, Philadelphia, Pennsylvania 19140

Enzymatic methyl modification of preformed proteins is a pervasive biochemical reaction occurring in both eukaryotes and prokaryotes (1-3). Proteins from many cell types are modified by specific methyltransferases, generally at the nucleophilic atoms such as nitrogen and oxygen of side chains. The methyl donor for the reaction is a sulfonium cation of S-adenosyl-L-methionine (SAM) and the demethylated product is S-adenosyl-L-homocysteine (SAH). It is known that lysyl, arginyl and histidyl residues are N-methylated and free carboxyl groups are O-methylated. Three methylating enzymes have been identified and characterized in our laboratory.

I) S-Adenosylmethionine:protein-arginyl N-methyltransferase, (EC.2.1.1.23; Protein methylase I): The enzyme methylates the guanidino group of arginine residues and yields $N^G$-monomethylarginine; $N^G,N^G$-dimethylarginine and $N^G,N'^G$-dimethylarginine on acid-hydrolysis of the protein.

II) S-Adenosylmethionine:protein-carboxyl O-methyltransferase,(EC.2.1.1.24; Protein methylase II): The enzyme methyl esterifies the carboxyl groups of aspartyl or glutamyl residues in the protein yielding carboxyl methyl esters of the respective amino acids.

III) S-Adenosylmethionine:protein-lysyl N-methyltransferase,(EC.2.1.1.42; Protein methylase III): $\varepsilon$-Amino groups of lysine residues are methylated and the products on acid-hydrolysis of the protein are $N^\varepsilon$-mono, $N^\varepsilon$-di- and $N^\varepsilon$-trimethyllysine.

These means to alter protein primary structure may be economical from the standpoint of cellular energetics, since the expenditure of ATP and GTP for the synthesis of polypeptide chains is conserved and yet proteins of different structure are formed. From the structure-functional relationship of protein this minor modification at the post-synthetic phase of protein may facilitate the rapidity of response and may be involved in more subtle functions of cellular metabolism such as occur in the central nervous system (CNS). This paper will review recent developments on protein methylation systems which are relevant only to the CNS, emphasizing protein methylase I and II. Among many findings, included are the properties and the levels of protein methyltransferases in the brain tissue as well as enzymatic methylation

37

of polypeptides originating from the CNS.  Although the role of protein methylation
on the physiology of the CNS is not clear at this time, there is sufficient evidence
which indicates perspectives on protein methylation.

## GENERAL CONSIDERATIONS

Close relationship of brain metabolism and protein methylating systems emerged from
several lines of observations:

a) Rat brain has the highest amount of protein methylases among the tissues.  The
   changes of the enzyme level in the brain is a function of age, showing parallel
   increase of protein methylase II activity during brain development, but decrease
   of the activities of methylase I and III during the same period (4).

b) Presence of methylarginine is found at Res-107 of encephalitogenic basic myelin
   protein, one of the major structural proteins of the CNS (5,6).

c) Methylated lysine and arginine residues are found in the acid hydrolyzate of
   cerebral proteins (7).

d) Substantial amount of endogenous substrate for protein methylase II was found
   only from the posterior and anterior pituitary glands, indicating in vivo methyl
   esterification of pituitary polypeptide hormones in the glands (8).

Although protein methylases I, II and III have been often studied as one family of
methyltransferases because of their similarity in enzymatic reactions, each reaction
nevertheless has its unique characteristics in terms of products, endogenous methyl
acceptor substrate, and, probably, physiological roles.

## PROTEIN-ARGINYL METHYLATION

A. Protein methylase I (S-Adenosylmethionine:protein-arginyl N-methyltransferase,
   EC.2.1.1.23).

Protein methylase I transfers methyl groups of SAM to arginyl residues in the protein substrate.  The enzyme was initially discovered in calf thymus during the course
of enzymatic methylation of lysyl residues (9).  Recently about 120-fold purification of the enzyme has been achieved from calf brain cytosol (10).  The optimum pH
of the reaction is 7.2 and the pI value is 5.1.  The $K_m$ values for SAM and an encephalitogenic basic myelin protein are $7.6 \times 10^{-6}$M and $7.1 \times 10^{-5}$M respectively,
and $K_i$ value for SAH is $2.62 \times 10^{-6}$M.  Although the enzymatic products after hydrolysis of the methylated protein are $N^G$, $N^G$-di(asymmetric)(asDMArg); $N^G$, $N'^G$-di
(symmetric)(sDMArg) and $N^G$-monomethylarginine (MMArg), the ratio of the three
methylarginine derivatives catalyzed by the enzyme preparations at different stages
of purification remains unchanged at 40:5:55 respectively, indicating that a single
enzyme is involved in the synthesis of the three arginine derivatives.  The kinetic
mechanism of the enzyme reaction with the purified enzyme is a sequential ordered

Bi-Bi mechanism in that SAM is the first substrate bound to the enzyme, and SAH is the last product released from the enzyme.

The enzyme is found predominantly in the cytosolic fraction of tissues; 70% of total enzyme activity can be recovered from 105,000xg supernatant of calf brain.  Since both encephalitogenic basic protein and histones are in vivo substrates for the enzyme and histone is a nuclear protein, a question was raised whether or not different substrates are methylated by specific enzymes.  Jones and Carnegie found no evidence for the existence of two enzymes specific for the methylation of myelin protein and histone (11), but Miyake reported two forms of methylases from rat brain, one for myelin basic protein and the other for histone (12).  The myelin protein methylating activity in the cell sap fraction was shown to increase during myelination, while histone methylase from the nuclear fraction was highest at birth with no correlation with the process of myelination.  In this connection, it might be interesting to speculate a possibility of a third enzyme which specifically methylates arginyl residues of heterogenous RNA-binding protein recently reported by Boffa et al.(13).

B.  Encephalitogenic Myelin Basic Protein as a Endogenous Substrate

The first evidence that one of the endogenous substrates for protein methylase I in the rat brain is the encephalitogenic basic protein of myelin sheath came from the sequence study of the protein.

The microheterogeneity of purified protein observed during electrophoresis (14) was due to the presence of the mixture of mono- and dimethylarginine at Res-107.  Analyzing the proportion of the two different degrees of the methylated arginine, Brostoff and Eyler (5) found that the Res-107 of bovine myelin protein is a mixture of sDMArg and MMArg with the ratio of 0.2:0.4-0.8 mole.  On the other hand Deibler and Marteson (15) found an approximately same amount of sDMArg and MMArg.  Furthermore, MMArg was not detected in the frog myelin and none of the methyl arginines were found in carp myelin.  Although the ratio of occurrence of methyl arginine derivatives in the myelin protein varies depending on the source of species, methylarginine in the protein is characterized by the absence of asDMArg, in contrast to the high amount of asDMArg in heterogenous nuclear ribonucleoprotein (HnRNP) fractions from rat liver (13).

When the occurrence of methylarginine in encephalitogenic basic protein was first reported as the enzymatic product (48), an exiciting speculation was put forward to explain the modification as a mechanism by which myelin sheath maintains its structural integrity.  The hypothesis was strengthened by the fact that methyl introduction to the guanidino group of arginine increases hydrophobicity of the residue, thus favoring stabilization of double chain structure of the protein which is assisted by Pro-Pro-Pro sequence: the (proline)$_3$ sequence that forms a sharp bend in the polypeptide double-chain structure occurs 5 amino acid residues away from that of methylarginine (5). Furthermore, Res-107 methylarginine also occurs close to the principal encephalitogenic determinant composed of residues 111-121 in the protein, and that determinant contains the sole tryptophan residue which has been postulated to be the receptor site for 5-hydroxy tryptamine (6).

An attempt was made to correlate myelination and the enzyme activity which methylates arginine residue of the myelin basic protein. However, brain protein methylase I of the rat did not show any significant changes in activity during active myelination (11,16), nor did this occur in jimpy mice, a mutant strain known to have degenerative myelination (4).

## PROTEIN-CARBOXYL METHYL ESTERIFICATION

A. Protein Methylase II (S-Adenosylmethionine:protein-carboxyl 0-methyltransferase, EC.2.1.1.24)

Protein methylase II methylates (esterifies) free carboxyl groups in substrate polypeptides with SAM as the methyl donor. The reaction was once described as by "methanol-forming enzyme" (17) and it was thought that SAM was hydrolyzed to yield methanol and SAH. However, Liss et al. (18) and Kim and Paik (19) have reported an enzyme which methylates protein with SAM. The methylated protein liberated a volatile methyl compound which was identified as methanol. Because the same substrate and hydrolytic end product were involved in both enzyme systems, comparative studies on these two enzymes were carried out. Based on the comparison of the various properties of the two enzymes and the unstable nature of the enzymatic products, it was concluded that the two enzymes are identical (20).

The enzyme has been highly purified from various mammalian organs by means of ion exchange and molecular sieve chromatography (20,21), and by affinity chromatography (22). In the last case, the product of the reaction, SAH, covalently linked to Sepharose-4B proved to be an effective binder for protein methylase II at pH 6.2, and allowed for specific removal of the enzyme with a buffer containing SAM. Using this affinity chromatography, the enzyme has been purified 3,000-fold from the calf brain. Heterogeneity of the enzyme was found with respect to molecular size as well as pI value, although the predominant form of the enzyme has a molecular weight of 25,000 daltons as estimated by molecular sieve chromatography (21).

Initial velocity and product inhibition studies with the purified enzyme showed the kinetic mechanism to be sequential rapid equilibrium random Bi-Bi in which the rate limiting step is the interconversion of the ternary complex of substrate proteins, SAM and the enzyme (23). The limiting Michaelis constant for SAM is $0.87 \times 10^{-6}$M, and $K_i$ values for SAH and adenosine are $1 \times 10^{-6}M$ and $1.2 \times 10^{-3}M$ respectively. $K_m$ values for various substrate proteins or peptides were also determined (Table 1).

Table 1    MICHAELIS CONSTANT VALUES OF PROTEIN METHYLASE II TOWARD VARIOUS SUBSTRATES

| Substrate | $K_m$ ($\mu$M) | Source of enzyme |
|---|---|---|
| Follicle-stimulating hormone (porcine) | 7.7 | calf thymus |
| Neurophysin (bovine) | 15.5 | bovine post. pituitary |
| Luteinizing hormone (sheep) | 50 | calf thymus |
| γ-globulin (bovine) | 46 | bovine post. pituitary |
| Ovalbumin | 54 | bovine post. pituitary |
| Serum albumin (bovine) | 70 | bovine post. pituitary |
| Ribonuclease (bovine pancreas) | 310 | bovine post. pituitary |
| Ribonuclease (bovine pancreas) | 400 | calf thymus |
| S-peptide (bovine panc. ribonuclease) | 2000 | calf thymus |
| Pentapeptide (Phe-Asp-Ala-Ser-Val) | 3200 | calf thymus |
| Heptapeptide (Lys-Glu-Thr-Ala-Ala-Ala-Lys) | 3600 | calf thymus |

Among the many methyl acceptors, follicle-stimulating hormone (23) and neurophysin (24) have been found to have the highest affinity to the enzyme. Using various chain length polypeptides as methyl acceptors, it was found that the $K_m$ values for the polypeptide substrates are inversely correlated with the length of the peptides; the shorter the peptide, the larger the $K_m$ values, while $V_{max}$ is related to the number of potential methyl acceptor sites in the molecule (25).

The enzyme is localized in the cytosol fraction of most mammalian tissues except brain, in which only 60% of the enzyme is in the cytosol (22); the remaining enzyme is synaptosome-associated or membrane-bound (26). Studies on the axonal transportation of the enzyme by a ligation of the rat sciatic nerve indicated that the enzyme accumulated proximal to the ligation, although the rate was slow (26).

B.   Endogenous Substrate for Protein Methylase II

The main drawback in understanding the physiological role of the enzyme is the unidentified nature of its in vivo substrate. This difficulty is the result of the instability of the enzymatic products, which are easily hydrolyzable in mild alkali (27). As shown in Fig. 1, the half-life of oxidized ribonuclease methyl ester prepared enzymatically is 25 min at pH 7.1, and 4 min at 8.6, at 37°C. Therefore, under physiological conditions, the endogenous protein methyl ester may not be present in a stable form. Isolation of such an ester from any biological materials

S. Kim, P. Galletti and K. Paik

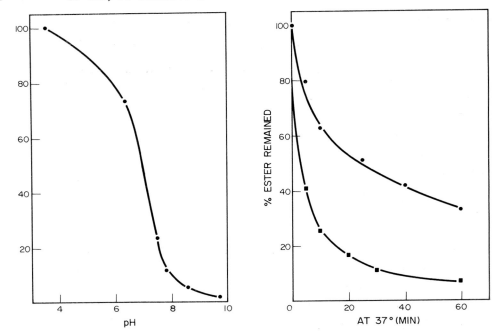

Fig. 1   The rate of hydrolysis of methyl esterified oxidized ribonuclease by protein methylase II.   Left, the hydrolysis was carried out at 37°C for 30 min at the indicated pHs.   Right, ●———●,
in 0.1 M Na phosphate pH 7.1; o———o, in 0.1 M tris-HCl pH 8.6
(27).

by routine protein isolation methods may not be successful.   To overcome this difficulty, the enzyme activity was measured with and without addition of exogenous
substrate (8).   If an enzyme preparation is saturated in respect to the protein substrate, an addition of exogenous substrate should not further increase the enzyme
activity.   Therefore, the ratio of exogenous over endogenous activity should be
close to unity.   Examining various parts of rabbit brain, it was found that posterior
and anterior pituitary glands had lower ratios, indicating high endogenous substrate
(8).   That the endogenous substrates in the pituitary glands are the various polypeptide hormones was further supported by the in vitro methylation of the polypeptides (28) and also by pituitary organ culture experiments (29).

Synthesis of endogenous substrate polypeptides in the hypothalamus and anterior
pituitary gland were shown during the hypothalamo-neuro-hypophysial complex in organ culture (29).   Increased endogenous enzyme activity was observed at the 7th day
of the culture in hypothalamus and at the 12th day in the anterior pituitary gland
and persisted for 3 weeks.

1.   Methyl Esterification of Pituitary Polypeptides

Anterior pituitary polypeptides:   The extent of methyl esterification of anterior pituitary polypeptide hormones was studied in the presence of excess amounts of purified calf brain protein methylase II and SAM but limiting amounts of methyl acceptor substrate. The methylated peptide was conveniently separated by molecular sieve chromatography (Fig 2).

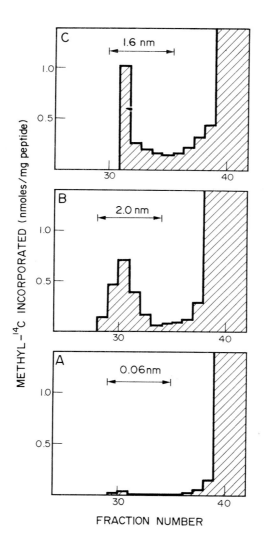

Fig. 2  Enzymatic methyl esterification of ovine β-lipotropin. The methylated lipotropin was separated by a column of Sephadex G-10 (0.6 x 70 cm) which was equilibrated with 0.1 N acetic acid. A, 0 min incubation; B, 30 min incubation; C, 60 min incubation.

As shown in Table 2, degree of esterification greatly depends on the polypeptide used for the reaction.   It may be noted that lutropin and adrenocorticotropin (ACTH)

TABLE II   ENZYMATIC METHYL ESTERIFICATION OF PITUITARY POLYPEPTIDES

| Methyl Acceptor Polypeptides | Period incubation (min) | Amount (nmoles) | $^{14}CH_3$-incorporation | |
|---|---|---|---|---|
| | | | nmoles | mole % |
| lutropin | 15 | 32.8 | 2.15 | 6.6 |
| lutropin-α | " | 62.5 | 2.58 | 4.1 |
| lutropin-β | " | 62.5 | 0.25 | 0.4 |
| prolactin | 30 | 47.8 | 0.18 | 0.4 |
| human somatotropin | " | 43.5 | 0.34 | 0.8 |
| β-LPH | " | 110 | 2.00 | 1.8 |
| β-EP | 60 | 309 | 0.28 | 0.09 |
| ACTH | " | 178 | 8.55 | 4.8 |
| α1-17-ACTH | " | 330 | 0.55 | --- |

are the best acceptors for the methylation.   That β-lipotropin (β-LPH) was a good methyl acceptor and β-endorphin (β-EP) was not suggests that the methyl acceptor portion of lipotropin is probably situated in the N-terminal segment of the molecule (30).   Most noteworthy is the methyl esterification of lutropin: while the lutropin-α-subunit accepted 4.1 mole % of methyl groups, the β-subunit was almost devoid of the accepting activity.   It can therefore be assumed that 6.6 mole % incorporation in the lutropin molecule were mostly due to the α-subunit, since both subunits have similar molecular weight (31).

The time course of methylation was also studied: Methylation peaks at 15 min with lutropin and at 30 min with prolactin (Fig. 3).   These peaks are followed by rather rapid fall in the incorporation of methyl group upon continuous incubation at 37°. At the end of 2 hours incubation, about 3/4 of the previously incorporated methyl groups were lost.   This is most likely due to a de-esterification reaction which was progressing simultaneously (see also Fig. 1).   Therefore, methyl incorporation shown in Fig. 3 at any given time is a sum of two reactions, i.e., enzymatic esterification and chemical de-esterification, although interplay of these two reaction mechanisms is not yet clear.

Posterior Pituitary Polypeptides:   Since the major protein in the posterior pituitary gland, neurophysin, is a good substrate for protein methylase II and has been known as a carrier protein for vasopressin and oxytocin, the effect of methyl esterification of neurophysin was studied for its binding capacity to vasopressin (32). The results indicated that the ability of agarose-coupled (8-lysine) vasopressin to bind modified and unmodified neurophysin was similar.   However, it was of great

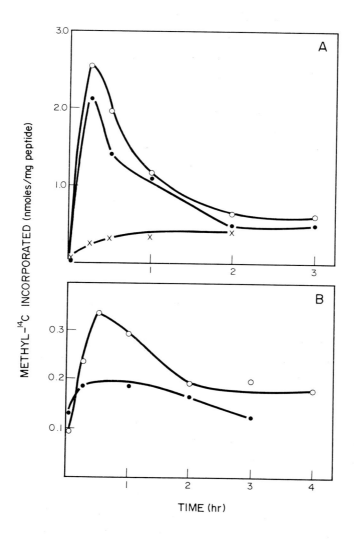

Fig. 3  Effect of methyl esterification of pituitary polypeptides.
A, ●——●, lutropin; o——o, lutropin-α-subunit; x——x, lutropin
β-subunit.
B, ●——●, prolactin; o——o, human somatotropin.

interest to observe that the rate of methyl esterification of neurophysin was influenced by non-methyl acceptor peptides.  While Edgar and Hope (24) observed a 35%
increase in the rate of the neurophysin I methylation by vasopressin, Diliberto et
al. observed an increase in neurophysin II methylation by oxytocin, vasopressin and
methionyl-tyrosyl-phenylalanineamide (33).  This increase may be the result of a
hormone-induced conformational change of neurophysin to which the enzyme exhibited

a greater affinity.

## 2. Methyl Esterification of Membrane Proteins

Exocytosis: It has been known that the negative surface potential of the catechol-amine-containing vesicle is derived from carboxyl groups of protein in the membrane, and during exocytosis the vesicle and plasma membrane fuse for discharge of the intravesicular products. An attractive hypothesis explaining the fusion process is an involvement of protein methylase II to neutralize the negative charge by enzymatic esterification of membrane protein. Thus, the possible role of protein methylase II in excitation-secretion coupling of chromaffin vesicle in the adrenal medulla was examined (34). Experimental results to support this hypothesis are: 1) of the various subcellular fractions of the adrenal medulla, the catecholamine-containing chromaffin vesicle has the highest concentration of substrate(s) for the enzyme, 2) adrenal medulla has several times higher specific enzyme activity than the adrenal cortex, and 3) carboxyl methylation of proteins in intact vesicles resulted in stripping of methylated proteins from the membranes.

Erythrocyte Membrane Proteins: Recently it was found that membrane proteins from the erythrocyte ghost serve as good methyl acceptors for protein methylase II (35). The methyl esterification is highly selective to the protein Bands 3 ($M_r$=97,000), 4 ($M_r$= 75,000) and 4.5 ($M_r$=48,000) as identified by sodium dodecyl sulfate-polyacrylamide gel electrophoresis. Although the biological implication of this membrane methylation is not known, in view of an important erythrocyte function, the modification might play a role in the membrane function.

Bacterial Chemotaxis: The interesting and exciting avenue of protein methylation and chemotaxis has been developed from an unexpected field of research, bacterial genetics. In 1969, Adler found that methionine was essential for chemotaxis of bacteria and methionine-starved auxotrophs did not show the ability for chemotaxis (36). Subsequently, the methionine requirement was shown to be for SAM (37). Using chemotactic mutants of E. coli and Salmonella typhimurium, methyl esterification of cytoplasmic membrane protein ($M_r$=62,000) has been shown to be affected by chemoattractants (38). Furthermore, the protein methylase that is responsible for the methylation of the membrane protein has been shown to be missing in the non-chemotactic mutant indicating the methylase as the cheR gene product (39). It is, therefore, proposed that methylation of cytoplasmic membrane is involved in bacterial sensing motion, although the relationship between the methylation and the rotation of the flagella which controls the rate of the bacterial motility is not known.

Mammalian Chemotaxis: Recently methyl esterification of leukocytes has also been investigated in relation to chemotaxis (40). Neutrophils isolated from peritoneal exudates posess chemotactic responsiveness. Upon incubation of the cell with the chemotactic peptide, Met-Leu-Phe, 2-3 fold increase in protein methyl-ester formation is observed in the neutrophil with a peak methylation at 30 sec after the addition of the tripeptide.  This finding suggests that methyl esterification of neutrophil protein (probably the chemotactic receptor in the membrane) mediated by the chemoattractant generated a signal for leukocyte motion.

PROTEIN-LYSYL METHYLATION

A. Protein Methylase III (S-adenosylmethionine:protein-lysyl N-methyltransferase EC.2.1.1.43).

Protein methylase III catalyzes transmethylation of the methyl group from SAM to lysyl residues of certain proteins.  The presence of the enzyme was originally demonstrated in calf thymus nuclei yielding mono- and dimethyl lysine on hydrolysis of the methylated nuclear protein (41).  In spite of the potential importance of the presence of methylated lysine in histones and many contractile proteins (42), the enzyme has not been purified successfully.  This is mainly due to the exclusive localization of the enzyme in nuclei where the enzyme is most likely complexed with other macromolecules such as DNA and chromosomal proteins.  The enzyme was solubilized from the calf thymus nuclei (43) and was recently purified from rat brain (44). The partially purified chromatin-bound enzyme methylates histones H3 and H4.  The ratio of $N^\epsilon$-mono-:$N^\epsilon$-di-:$N^\epsilon$-trimethyllysine in histone H3 was 1.8:1.0:0.45 and the ratio of $N^\epsilon$-mono:$N^\epsilon$-dimethyllysine in H4 was 0.7:1.0.  SAH is a competitive inhibitor with $K_i$ value of $6 \times 10^{-6}$M.  Interestingly, protein methylase III from Krebs 2 ascites chromatin catalyzes the formation of only $N^\epsilon$-trimethyllysine (45).

B. Brain Histone Methylation.

Matured brain cells do not divide, but develop rapidly during the first few days of life.  Thus, under the premise that histones might regulate gene action, side chain methylation of brain histone has been studied.  Protein methylase III activity was studied with histone as the methyl acceptor during rat brain development (4,16). When protein methylase III activity was measured in the presence of histone as substrate (4,16) the activity per cell increased rapidly reaching a peak of about 10 days after birth and thereafter decreased.  Consistent with this finding, the ability of brain histones to accept methyl group also decreased during aging (46), suggesting that brain histone methylation is an irreversible reaction and that additional methylation may not take place once they are methylated.

Tissue heterogeneity of histone methylation was also studied by Deurre and his coworkers (47).  The distribution of methyl groups on the lysyl residues in the $F_3$ and $F_{2a1}$ histones from the different organs, such as cerebrum, cerebellum, liver, kidney and thymus was similar, indicating no apparent tissue specificity associated with specific pattern of histone lysine methylation.

## CONCLUDING REMARKS

Recent advances in the methylation of proteins presented in this review illustrate as yet fully unexplored post-translational modification of protein in the CNS. Three well characterized protein methylases, I, II and III are discussed in terms of their natural substrates and enzymology.

Protein methylase II which forms protein-methyl ester needs particular attention because of its formation of an inherently unstable ester and neutraliation of negative charge by methyl esterification. Natural endogenous substrates for this reaction appear to be various pituitary polypeptide hormones and certain membrane proteins from adrenal chromaffin vesicles and erythrocyte ghosts. Increasing interest in protein carboxyl methylation focuses on chemotactic action both in prokaryotic bacteria and in mammalian leukocytes.

Although various model systems have been used to understand the physiological role of protein methylation, each system bears its own exciting speculations. At present, these speculations are at the embryonic stages; therefore further investigations are required for finalization of these hypotheses. Nevertheless, it should be pointed out that a common ground for these hypotheses lies in the possibliity that methylation may alter the interaction of molecules between methylated residue and surroundings, since introduction of a methyl group to the side chains is known to increase hydrophobicity and charge alteration. Therefore, these protein structural modifications will induce functional modifications and may contribute subtle changes in cellular metabolism by molecular interactions including hormone-receptor, hormone-carrier, protein-lipid and protein-DNA interactions. In any event, whatever the interacting molecule may be, the process probably is the earliest biochemical event to which surrounding molecules respond.

## REFERENCES

1.  Paik, W.K. and Kim, S. Science 174, 114 (1971).

2.  Paik, W.K. and Kim, S. Adv. Enzymol. 42, 227 (1975).

3.  Kim, S. in The Biochemistry of Adenosylmethionine, Eds. F. Salvatore, E. Borek, V. Zappia, H.G. Williams-Ashman and F. Schlenk, Columbia Univ. Press, N.Y., 415 (1977).

4.  Paik, W.K. and Kim, S. Biochim. Biophys. Acta 313, 181 (1973).

5.  Brostoff, S. and Eylar, E.H. Proc. Nat. Acad. Sci. U.S.A. 68, 765 (1971).

6.  Carnegie, P.R. Nature 229, 25 (1971).

7.  Kakimoto, Y. Biochim. Biophys. Acta 243, 31 (1971).

8.   Kim, S., Wasserman, L., Lew, B. and Paik, W.K. J. Neurochem. 24, 625 (1975).

9.   Paik, W.K. and Kim, S. J. Biol. Chem. 243, 2108 (1968).

10.  Lee, W.H., Kim, S. and Paik, W.K. Biochemistry 16, 78 (1977).

11.  Jones, G.M. and Carnegie, P.R. J. Neurochem. 23, 1231 (1974).

12.  Miyake, M. J. Neurochem. 24, 909 (1975).

13.  Boffa, L.C., Karn, J., Vidali, C.T. and Allfrey, V.G. Biochem. Biophys. Res. Comm. 74, 969 (1977).

14.  Martenson, R.E., Deibler, G.E. and Kier, M.W. J. Biol. Chem. 244, 4261 (1969).

15.  Deibler, G.E.  and Martenson, R.E. J. Biol. Chem. 248, 2387 (1973).

16.  Paik, W.K. and Kim, S. Biochem. Biophys. Res. Comm. 46, 933 (1972).

17.  Axelrod, J. and Daly, J. Science 150, 892 (1965).

18.  Liss, M., Maxam, A.M. and Cuprak, L. J. Biol. Chem. 244, 1617 (1969).

19.  Kim, S. and Paik, W.K. J. Biol. Chem. 245, 1806 (1970).

20.  Kim, S. Arch. Biochem. Biophys. 157, 476 (1973)

21.  Kim, S. Arch. Biochem. Biophys. 161, 652 (1974).

22.  Kim, S., Nochumson, S., Chin, W. and Paik, W.K. Anal. Biochem. 84, 415 (1978).

23.  Jamaluddin, M., Kim, S. and Paik, W.K. Biochemistry 14, 694 (1975).

24.  Edgar, D.H. and Hope, D.B. J. Neurochem. 26, 1 (1976)

25.  Jamaluddin, M., Kim, S. and Paik, W.K. Biochemistry 15, 3077 (1976)

26.  Diliberto, E.J., Jr., and Axelrod, J. J. Neurochem. 26, 1159 (1976).

27.  Kim, S. and Paik, W.K. Experientia 32, 982 (1976).

28.  Diliberto, E.J., Jr. and Axelrod, J. Proc. Natl. Acad. Sci. 71, 1701 (1974).

29.  Kim, S., Pearson, D. and Paik, W.K. Biochem. Biophys. Res. Comm. 67, 448 (1975).

30.  Li, C.H. and Chung, D. Nature 260, 622 (1976).

31.  Sairam, M.R., Papkoff, H. and Li, C.H. Biochem. Biophys. Res. Comm. 48, 530 (1972).

32.  Edgard, D.H. and Hope, D.B. FEBS LETTERS 49, 145 (1974).

33.  Diliberto, E.J., Jr., Axelrod, J. and Chaiken, I.M. Biochem. Biophys. Res. Comm. 73, 1063 (1976).

34.  Diliberto, E.J., Jr., Viveros, O.H. and Axelrod, J. Proc. Natl. Acad. Sci. USA, 73, 4050 (1976).

35.  Galletti, P., Paik, W.K. and Kim, S. Fed. Proc. in press (1978).

36.  Adler, J. Science 166, 1588 (1969).

37.  Aswad, D. and Koshland, D.E., Jr. J. Mol. Biol. 97, 207 (1975).

38.  Kort, E.N., Goy, M.F., Larsen, S.H. and Adler, J. Proc. Natl. Acad. Sci. USA 72, 3939 (1975).

39.  Springer, W.R. and Koshland, D.E., Jr. Proc. Natl. Acad. Sci. USA 74, 533 (1977).

40.  O'Dea, R.F., Viveros, O.H., Axelrod, J., Aswanikumar, S., Schiffmann, E. and Coccoran, B.A. Nature 272, 462 (1978).

41.  Kim, S. and Paik, W.K. J. Biol. Chem. 240, 4629 (1965).

42.  Huszan, G. J. Biol. Chem., 247 4057 (1972).

43.  Paik, W.K. and Kim, S. J. Biol. Chem. 245, 6010 (1970).

44.  Wallwork, J.C., Quick, D.P. and Duerre, J.A. J. Biol. Chem. 252, 5977 (1977).

45.  Burdon, R.H. and Gaven, E.V. Biochim. Biophys. Acta. 232, 371 (1971).

46.  Lee, C. and Duerre, J.A. Nature 251, 240 (1974).

47.  Duerre, J.A. and Chakrabarty, S. J. Biol. Chem. 250, 8457 (1975).

48.  Baldwin, G.S. and Carnegie, P.R. Science 171, 579 (1971).

# The Relation Between Folate and Adenosylmethionine Metabolism in Brain

## Anthony J. Turner, Andrew G. M. Pearson and Robert J. Mason

Department of Biochemistry, University of Leeds, 9 Hyde Terrace,
Leeds LS2 9LS, England

"Adenosyl methionine is the sole methyl donor in all methyl
transfer reactions, except those resulting in the biosynthesis of methionine."

Giulio Cantoni, 1952

The addition or removal of a non-carbon group from biological compounds is a common
metabolic occurrence and, of the groups involved in such transfer reactions, carbon
dioxide is the species most often used. However, where the transfer of one-carbon
groups at different oxidation states is required, the intracellular pool of folates
is called into play. Derivatives of tetrahydrofolate ($FH_4$) function as cofactors
in a variety of biologically important transformations including nucleotide metabolism, amino acid metabolism and the biosynthesis of methyl groups. The question
posed in this review is whether $N^5$-methyl FH4 ($CH_3FH_4$) functions only in the provision of methyl groups for methionine biosynthesis or whether it may act directly
in neurotransmitter methylation processes in brain.

ENZYMOLOGY OF FOLATE METABOLISM IN BRAIN

The folic acid molecule is composed of a pterin moiety linked via a p-aminobenzoyl
group to one or more glutamate residues (Fig.1). Naturally occuring folates may
differ from one another in three major respects: the nature and position of one-
carbon substituents, the state of oxidation of the pterin nucleus and the number of
glutamate residues present in the molecule. Folic acid itself is reduced via 7,8-
dihydrofolic acid to the active form of the vitamin (5,6,7,8-tetrahydrofolate) in
a reaction catalysed by dihydrofolate reductase. Dihydrofolic acid is also formed
as a result of the thymidylate synthase reaction, and must likewise be re-converted
to tetrahydrofolate by the action of dihydrofolate reductase. A detailed discussion
of the pathways of folate metabolism has been given elsewhere (1).

The major circulating form of folates is $CH_3FH_4$ (Fig. 1), which occurs predominantly
in a protein-bound form in blood (2) and can be concentrated into brain by a satur-

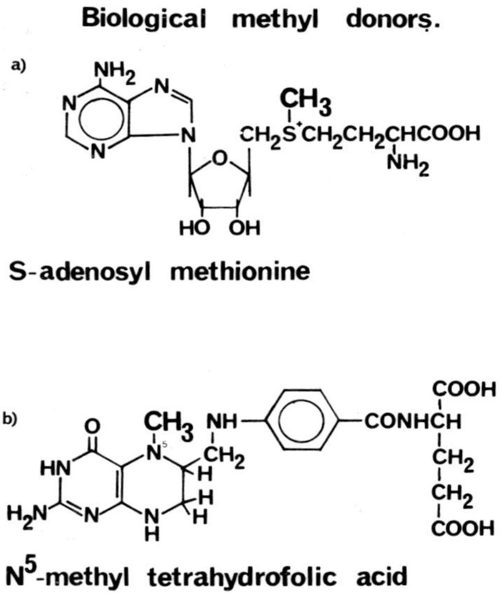

**Biological methyl donors.**

S-adenosyl methionine

$N^5$-methyl tetrahydrofolic acid

Fig. 1.   Comparison of the structures of the biological methyl donors
(a) SAM and (b) $N^5$-methyltetrahydrofolate ($CH_3FH_4$)

able uptake process with a Michaelis constant for transport of 18 nM (3).  It has
been suggested that the requirement for uptake of the reduced form of folates, maintained even in folate-deficiency states (4), is essential because brain tissue lacks
dihydrofolate reductase activity (5).  However, re-investigation of the ability of
nervous tissue to reduce dihydrofolate has shown that the enzyme is present, albeit
in low concentration, in rat and rabbit brain (6-8).  We have detected methotrexate-
sensitive dihydrofolate reductase activity in the cytosol of ox brain at a level of
0.23 nmol/min/mg protein (Table 1). .Blood contamination has been excluded as the
source of the reductase (8).  The brain enzyme can be distinguished from the related
enzyme dihydropteridine reductase by coenzyme specificity, sensitivity to methotrex-
ate and developmental characteristics (Table 1).  Dihydrofolate reductase shows
greatest activity in newborn rats when DNA synthesis is active (9), whereas dihydropteridine reductase activity increases with age (10).  Folates undoubtedly have
an important role to play in the maturation of the nervous system, and the ability
to regenerate the reduced form of the coenzyme may therefore be essential during
development.  However, the role of folate reductase in the adult brain is unclear,
although it may be involved in the formation of tetrahydrobiopterin, which is required as a cofactor for tryptophan and tyrosine hydroxylases (7,8).

TABLE 1    COMPARISON OF DIHYDROFOLATE REDUCTASE AND DIHYDROPTERIDINE
REDUCTASE FROM BRAIN AND LIVER

| Enzyme | Source | Reported activity (nmol/min/mg) | % Inhibition by 10 µM methotrexate | Neo-natal activity / adult activity |
|---|---|---|---|---|
| Dihydrofolate reductase | Brain (ox, rat, rabbit) | 0.05 - 0.33 | 100 | 2.6 |
| (EC 1.5.1.3) | Liver (ox, rat) | 1.8  - 5.7 | 100 | 2.2 |
| Dihydropteridine reductase | Brain (rat) | 32 - 80 | 25 | 0.31 |
| (EC 1.6.99.7) | Liver (rat, sheep) | 110 - 600 | 11* | - |

*Calculated from $K_i$ value of 38 µM (Ref. 11).

Data are compiled from Refs. 6-14 and Turner and Mason (unpublished).

Liver tissue possesses the ability to synthesize methionine from homocysteine using
either betaine or $CH_3FH_4$ as methyl donor and the relative contributions of the two
pathways may vary with dietary and hormonal status of the animal (15).   Early attempts to demonstrate the conversion of homocysteine to methionine in brain were
unsuccessful, possibly because of insufficient sensitivity of the method employed
(16).   However, brain tissue has now been shown to synthesize the methyl group of
methionine *de novo* using $CH_3FH_4$ as methyl donor (17).   Betaine apparently cannot
serve as methyl donor in brain (15), nor can the enzyme formiminotransferase contribute to the one-carbon pool in nervous tissue (18).   Serine probably provides the
major source of one-carbon units to the folate-pool in brain via serine hydroxymethyltransferase.   This reaction results in the formation of the intermediate methyl-
ene-$FH_4$ in which the one-carbon unit is at the oxidation level of formaldehyde.   Indeed methylene-$FH_4$ exists in equilibrium with $FH_4$ and free formaldehyde (dissociation constant - 31 µM at pH 7.2) (1).   Methylene-$FH_4$ may also be generated in brain
from glycine by the action of the intra-mitochondrial glycine cleavage complex (19).
A number of alternative metabolic routes are available to methylene-$FH_4$ including
oxidation, reduction and involvement in the synthesis of dTMP.   The central role of
methylene-$FH_4$ in folate metabolism is illustrated in Fig. 2.

The first committed step in the biosynthesis of adenosyl methionine required the
reduction of methylene-$FH_4$ to $CH_3FH_4$ in a reaction catalysed by methylene-$FH_4$ reductase (Fig. 3).   This enzyme preferentially uses NADPH as reductant (in contrast
to the bacterial enzyme), and is stimulated by FAD (20).   In the reverse direction

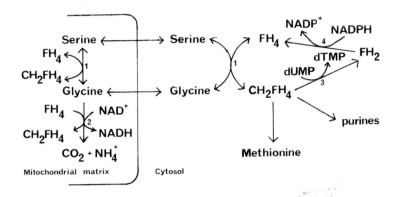

Fig. 2.  The central role of methylenetetrahydrofolate ($CH_2FH_4$) in one-
carbon metabolism. The transport of one-carbon units between
mitochondrial and cytosolic compartments may involve a serine/
glycine shuttle system (ref. 31). The enzyme systems referred
to are (1) serine hydroxymethyltransferase, (2) glycine cleavage complex, (3) thymidylate synthase and (4) dihydrofolate
reductase.

menadione may serve as oxidant and the enzyme also possesses an intrinsic NADPH-
dependent menadione reductase activity. The enzyme may therefore be assayed by
making use of any of the following reactions:

$$\text{Methylene-FH}_4 + \text{NADPH} + \text{H}^+ \longrightarrow \text{CH}_3\text{FH}_4 + \text{NADP}^+ \tag{1}$$

$$\text{CH}_3\text{FH}_4 + \text{Menadione} \longrightarrow \text{Methylene-FH}_4 + \text{Reduced menadione} \tag{2}$$

$$\text{Menadione} + \text{NADPH} + \text{H}^+ \longrightarrow \text{NADP}^+ + \text{Reduced menadione} \tag{3}$$

The menadione reductase assay (reaction 3) provides the most convenient procedure
for measuring enzyme activity, but is unsuitable for impure preparations because
brain contains large quantities of menadione reductase activity distinct from
methylene-FH$_4$ reductase. These two enzymes do, however, differ in molecular weight
and can be separated by gel filtration (21).

For crude extracts, the menadione dependent oxidation of $^{14}\text{CH}_3\text{FH}_4$ is generally
measured (reaction 2). The product ($^{14}$C-methylene-FH$_4$), which is in equilibrium
with FH$_4$ and H$^{14}$CHO, is quantified by forming the dimedone condensation product of
the formaldehyde (20). Since formaldehyde reacts readily with protein and other
tissue components, it is essential to check the recovery of the aldehyde by this
procedure, as well as the linearity of the assay with protein concentration.

Methylene-FH$_4$ reductase appears to be the rate-limiting and key regulatory enzyme
in the pathway to SAM since the latter compound inhibits the enzyme both in liver
and brain (17,20,22,23), probably by an allosteric mechanism. This inhibition is
partially relieved by SAH and therefore the ratio of the levels of these two com-

pounds is the important factor in regulating reductase activity and SAM biosynthesis
(20).  SAH may also control the activity of transmethylases (24) and it is noteworthy that the activity of SAH hydrolase in rat brain is only 10% of the levels in
liver (25).

The next step in SAM biosynthesis in the central nervous system (CNS) involves the
transfer of a methyl group from $CH_3FH_4$ to homocysteine to form methionine in a reaction requiring Vitamin $B_{12}$.  In cases of nutritional deficiency of $B_{12}$, tissue
levels of $CH_3FH_4$: homocysteine methyltransferase ($B_{12}$ transmethylase) are reduced
to such an extent that $CH_3FH_4$ levels increase above normal.  This phenomenon has
been termed the "methyl trap", because one-carbon groups become metabolically trap-
ped as $CH_3FH_4$ (1,26).  The methionine formed by the $B_{12}$-transmethylase is then ad-
enosylated by the enzyme methionine adenosyl transferase in a reaction requiring
ATP.  The interconversion of folate derivatives relevant to this assay are shown
in Fig. 3.  All the enzymes involved in this pathway are cytosolic with the except-

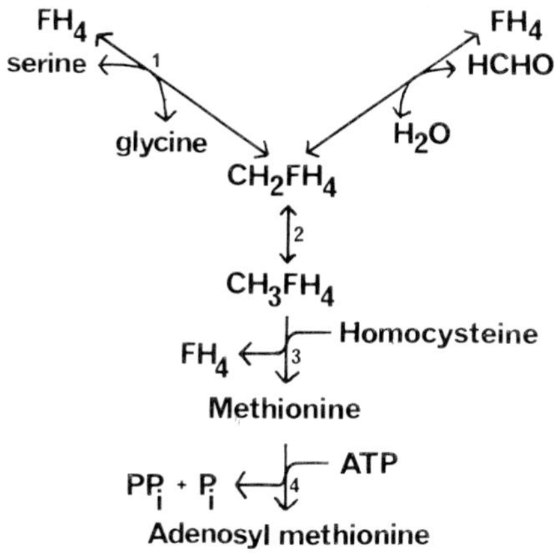

Fig. 3.   The pathway to SAM biosynthesis in brain.  The enzymes referred
          to are (1) serine hydroxymethyl transferase, (2) methylene-$FH_4$
          reductase, (3) $CH_3FH_4$ : homocysteine methyltransferase ($B_{12}$
          transmethylase) and (4) methionine adenosyltransferase.  The
          association of $FH_4$ with formaldehyde is presumed to be non-
          enzymic.

ion of serine hydroxymethyl transferase which occurs predominantly in the mitochondrial fraction of brain homogenates.  Reports on the proportion of this enzyme present in the cytosol vary from 1 to 30% (23,27-30).  Iso-enzymic forms of serine hydroxymethyltransferase in cytosolic and mitochondrial compartments would however pro-

vide a shuttle system for transport of one-carbon groups across the mitochondrial membrane (31) (see Fig. 2). Such a possibility requires further clarification. The levels of the relevant folate-enzymes in the CNS are listed in Table 2. The $B_{12}$

TABLE II.   LEVELS OF SOME FOLATE-ENZYMES INVOLVED IN SAM
             SYNTHESIS IN BRAIN

| Enzyme | E.C. Number | Activity range nmol/min/mg |
|---|---|---|
| Serine hydroxymethyltransferase | 2.1.2.1 | 0.27 - 0.77 |
| Methylene-FH$_4$ reductase | 1.1.1.68 | 0.028 - 0.042 |
| Methylene-FH$_4$ dehydrogenase | 1.5.1.5 | 0.86 - 5.15 |
| $B_{12}$ Transmethylase | 2.1.1.10 | 0.029 - 0.077 |
| Methionine adenosyl transferase | 2.5.1.6 | 0.053 - 0.06 |

The data are from a variety of species (mainly rat) and are taken from refs. 15, 17, 18, 27-30 and Turner and Mason (unpublished).

transmethylase is of comparable activity in brain and liver whereas the other enzymes are of considerably lower activity in brain. None of these enzymes has been obtained in a highly purified form from nervous tissue.

## METHYLATION PROCESSES IN TRANSMITTER METABOLISM

Adenosyl methionine functions in a wide range of transmethylation reactions, a number of which will be described in more detail in other chapters in this volume. SAM-dependent methylation processes are of particular importance in the biosynthesis and inactivation of neurotransmitter and hormonally active amines. For example, both the formation of melatonin and the inactivation of catecholamines involve O-methylation processes whereas the synthesis of adrenaline and the inactivation of histamine involve N-methylation reactions. In all cases SAM is the methyl donor.

A SAM-dependent enzyme capable of N-methylating a wide range of amines, and thus referred to as the "non-specific N-methyl transferase" was originally identified in lung tissue by Axelrod (32). This enzyme activity was subsequently reported to occur in several mammalian tissues, including brain, and was able to convert tryptaamine, to N,N-dimethyl tryptamine, a potent hallucinogen (33-35). This discovery lent weight to the "transmethylation hypothesis" of schizophrenia by which it was suggested that excessive methylation of transmitter amines could lead to the formation of endogenous hallucinogens (see Baldessarini, this volume). The role of methylating enzymes in brain function has been reviewed by Saavedra (36).

The non-specific N-methyl transferase was reported to be generally distributed throughout the brain and was located in the cytosol (35). However the activity was extremely low and was subject to inhibition by endogenous low molecular weight compounds (35), possibly peptide in nature (37). Re-examination of this N-methyl transferase has led to its occurrence in brain being questioned (38,39), although dimethyltryptamine has been shown to be formed *in vivo* in brain (40).

Because of doubts concerning the occurrence of non-specific N-methyl transferase in brain, Laduron examined the possibility of N-methylation of dopamine in brain (41, 42). He questioned the hypothesis that SAM is the only methyl donor in biological transmethylation reactions, apart from the conversion of homocysteine to methionine (43), and suggested that $CH_3FH_4$ may itself function as methyl donor to biogenic amines. Cantoni has pointed out that such a reaction would be of considerable interest mechanistically since $CH_3FH_4$ is about a thousand times less reactive than SAM towards nucleophiles such as amines (44). The structures of $CH_3FH_4$ and SAM are compared in Fig. 1.

A flurry of publications from independent laboratories apparently confirmed the original observations of Laduron and showed that $CH_3FH_4$ could act as methyl donor to catecholamines and indoleamines and that both N- and O-methylation could occur (45-47). The procedure adopted to measure activity involved the incubation of amine together with $^{14}CH_3FH_4$ and tissue extract. The radioactive products were then isolated by ion-exchange chromatography or solvent extraction and separated and identified by thin-layer chromatography. The folate-dependent methyltransferase was found to be present in various mammalian tissues and, in nervous tissue, was several times more active than the corresponding SAM-dependent methylation process. A folate-dependent methylation of uracil in transfer RNA has also been claimed (48), although the reaction was not examined in detail. A summary of the reported involvement of folate-derivatives in methylation reactions is provided in Table 3.

TABLE III.   REPORTED FOLATE-DEPENDENT METHYLATION PROCESSES

| Donor | Acceptor | Product | Ref. |
|---|---|---|---|
| Methylene-$FH_4$ | dUMP | dTMP | 1 |
| Methyl $FH_4$ | Homocysteine | Methionine | 1 |
| Methyl $FH_4$ | Dopamine | N-methyl dopamine | 41, 42 |
| Methyl $FH_4$ | Indoleamines | O- and N-methylated indoleamines | 42, 45, 46 |
| Methyl $FH_4$ (?) | tRNA | $m^5$ Uracil-tRNA | 48 |

The concept that $CH_3FH_4$ may function as a methyl donor to neurotransmitter amines provided a further boost to the transmethylation hypothesis of schizophrenia and the suggestion was made that an inborn error of folate metabolism might provide a biochemical explanation for certain types of psychoses (49). This metabolic lesion might have involved an excessive synthesis of methyl groups, a hyper-active transmethylating enzyme or a failure to degrade excess methyl donor. Because of the implications of this novel folate-dependent methylation we began to investigate the mechanism of this one-carbon transfer process.

## IDENTIFICATION OF THE PRODUCTS FORMED FROM FOLATE-DEPENDENT ONE-CARBON TRANSFER TO BIOGENIC AMINES

The first evidence suggesting that the folate-dependent methyl transferase may not catalyse a direct methylation of amines followed rapidly on the original reports from Laduron and others. Lin and Narasimhachari (50) examined the products formed by incubation of indolethylamines and rat brain extract with either $CH_3FH_4$ or SAM. They reported that when SAM was the methyl donor the products were isographic with standard 0- and N-methylated indolethylamine standards. When $CH_3FH_4$ was used as methyl donor however, the products corresponded to neither 0- nor N-methylated indolethylamines although the possibility of N-methylation of the indole ring could not be excluded. Mandel *et al.* (51) positively identified the product formed from $CH_3FH_4$ and **tryp**tamine as 1,2,3,4-tetrahydro-β-carboline ("tryptoline") and the structure of the product was confirmed by mass spectroscopy. These findings were independently confirmed by Wyatt *et al.* (52). When dopamine was the substrate, the product was shown not to be N-methyl dopamine as previously supposed but 6,7-dihydroxy-1,2,3,4-tetrahydroisoquinoline (53).

It has been known for some years that β-carboline and isoquinoline alkaloids can be formed from the parent amines by condensation with formaldehyde and this reaction has been exploited for the histochemical detection of catecholamines and indoleamines in brain (54). It then became apparent that the enzyme originally identified as a methyl transferase was capable of converting $CH_3FH_4$ to HCHO which could subsequently condense non-enzymically with amines to form isoquinoline or tryptoline alkaloids (Fig. 4). This explanation is consistent with the observation that di-N-methylated phenylethylamine derivatives were unable to accept radioactivity from $^{14}CH_3FH_4$ (42). That the reaction proceeds in two stages can be shown by the fact that significant amounts of product formation occurred when amine was added at the end of the incubation period (21). As the amine appears to play no direct role in the enzymic reaction, previously quoted kinetic constants for amine substrates (42, 45) have little significance. By what mechanism, then, is formaldehyde generated from $CH_3FH_4$ and does this process represent a novel reaction in folate metabolism in the CNS?

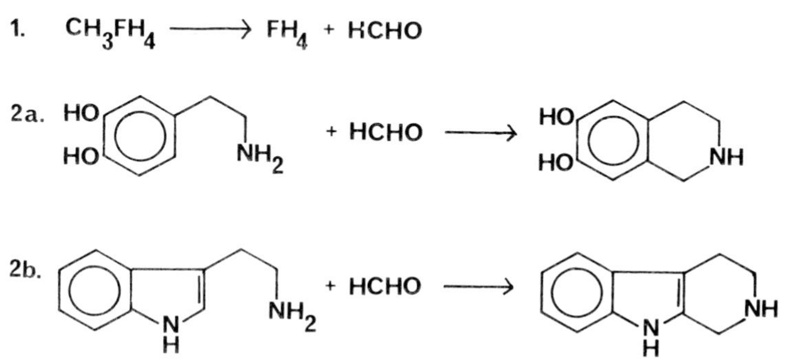

Fig. 4.  Route to the synthesis of tetrahydroisoquinoline and β-carboline alkaloids: (1) oxidation of methyl $FH_4$ to $FH_4$ and formaldehyde (2a) Pictet-Spengler condensation of dopamine with formaldehyde to form a tetrahydroisoquinoline, (2b) Pictet-Spengler
condensation of tryptamine with formaldehyde to form a tetrahy-
dro-β-carboline (tryptoline).

## THE ENZYME RESPONSIBLE FOR ONE-CARBON TRANSFER TO BIOGENIC AMINES

The significance of a "formaldehyde-forming enzyme" was unclear to us.  Formaldehyde is a reactive species and, if formed *in vivo*, its presence would be short-
lived since it could bind rapidly to tissue protein or other cell components (54) or
be oxidized by aldehyde dehydrogenases (55).  We therefore reasoned that the formation of formaldehyde could be a consequence of the action of methylene-$FH_4$ reductase present in the brain extract (see Fig. 3).  As stated above, although this
enzyme probably functions physiologically in the direction of $CH_3FH_4$ formation (56),
it may be assayed in the reverse direction by its ability to form methylene-$FH_4$
which exists in equilibrium with $FH_4$ and HCHO.  We therefore set out to establish
that methylene-$FH_4$ reductase and the putative dopamine methyl transferase activities
were catalyzed by a single protein.  The only published purification for this enzyme
from a mammalian source was from pig liver and this procedure was therefore adopted
(20).  We were unable to separate the two activities by ion-exchange chromatography,
gel filtration or isoelectric focusing (22).  Furthermore, the two activities were
similarly affected by a number of reagents: FAD caused a four-fold stimulation of
activity and the feedback regulator SAM blocked both activities.  Although we had
not obtained a homogenous preparation of the protein at this state we concluded
that the folate-dependent one-carbon transfer was probably mediated, in large part,
by the activity of the widely-distributed enzyme methylene-$FH_4$ reductase (22).  Similar conclusions have been reached by other authors (57,58) and moreover these two
enzyme  activities show a similar distribution pattern in rat brain (Table 4).

A. J. Turner, A. G. M. Pearson and R. J. Mason

TABLE IV.   REGIONAL DISTRIBUTION IN RAT BRAIN OF THE PURPORTED "DOPAMINE METHYL TRANSFERASE" AND METHYLENE-$FH_4$ REDUCTASE

| Brain region | Relative specific activity | |
| --- | --- | --- |
| | Dopamine $CH_3$-transferase | $CH_2$-$FH_4$ reductase |
| Corpus striatum | 1.00 | 1.00 |
| Lumbo-sacral cord | 0.83 | 0.84 |
| Hypothalamus | 0.70 | 0.73 |
| Corpora quadrigemini | 0.66 | 0.69 |
| Cerebellum | 0.66 | 0.78 |
| Medulla | 0.55 | 0.66 |
| Hippocampus | 0.44 | 0.48 |
| Occipital cortex | 0.39 | 0.52 |
| Frontal cortex | 0.37 | 0.61 |

Data taken from Hsu and Mandell (66) and Burton and Sallach (23).

More recently, we have sought to obtain additional evidence for the role of methylene-$FH_4$ as an intermediate in the synthesis of tetrahydroisoquinoline and β-carboline alkaloids. If the reaction occurs by the mechanism that we have proposed, then any reaction generating methylene-$FH_4$ should be capable of forming these alkaloids. One such reaction is that catalyzed by serine hydroxymethyl transferase:

$$\text{serine} + FH_4 \rightleftharpoons \text{glycine} + \text{methylene-}FH_4$$

To test whether the 3-carbon atom of serine could be transferred to biogenic amines with the concomitant formation of alicyclic alkaloids the following experiments were performed. Serine hydroxymethyl transferase was purified from ox liver by the method of Jones and Priest (59). The purification procedure involved a heat denaturation step followed by ion-exchange chromatography on CM-Sephadex and then affinity chromatography on folate-Sepharose. The final, purified product contained no detectable methylene-$FH_4$ reductase activity. A sample of the enzyme (0.05 units) was incubated at pH 7.4 with L-[3-$^{14}$C]serine, $FH_4$ and tryptamine for 30 mins at 30°C (for details, see legend to Table 5). Blank incubations were performed in the absence of $FH_4$ or by using enzyme that had been inactivated by boiling. After incubation, the reaction products were adjusted to pH 10, extracted into toluene, and separated by thin-layer chromatography. The results documented in Table 5 demonstrate that both serine hydroxymethyl transferase and methylene-$FH_4$ reductase can,

under appropriate conditions, convert an indoleamine to a compound with similar
chromatographic properties to a tryptoline alkaloid.

TABLE V.  TRYPTOLINE FORMATION MEDIATED BY SERINE HYDROXYMETHYL
          TRANSFERASE (SHMT) AND METHYLENE-FH$_4$ REDUCTASE

| Incubation | Enzyme | Radioactivity recovered as tryptoline (dpm) |
|---|---|---|
| 1 | SHMT (native) | 1500 |
| 2 | SHMT (denatured) | <30 |
| 3 | SHMT (-FH$_4$) | <30 |
| 4 | CH$_2$FH$_4$ Reductase (native) | 500 |
| 5 | CH$_2$FH$_4$ Reductase (denatured) | <30 |

SHMT (0.05 units) was incubated in a stoppered glass tube in a total vol. of 0.5
ml with: 30 µmol potassium phosphate buffer, pH 7.4; 0.1 µmol pyridoxal phosphate;
0.1 µmol L-[3-$^{14}$C]serine (0.5 µ Ci), 0.8 µmol FH$_4$ and 10 µmol tryptamine. Blank incubations were performed with denatured enzyme or in the absence of FH$_4$ (-FH$_4$).  Products extracted into toluene and separated by TLC on silica gel (butan-1-ol/acetic
acid/water) (60 : 30 : 10).  The incubations with CH$_3$FH$_4$ reductase were performed
in the presence of 0.5 µCi [$^{14}$C]-CH$_2$FH$_4$ and 10 µmol tryptamine HCl.

We have further sought to obtain methylene-FH$_4$ reductase from ox brain in a high
degree of purity in order to investigate more fully the role that SAM plays in the
regulation of this enzyme.  Conventional affinity resins, such as NADP-Sepharose
and 2'5'ADP-Sepharose did not bind methylene-FH$_4$ reductase.  We therefore turned to
the use of immobilized chlorotriazinyl dyes for the purification of the enzyme.  The
dye Cibacron Blue F3GH (Fig. 5) (the chromaphore of blue dextran) has been shown to
interact with a number of nucleotide-containing enzymes and has been used in their
purification (60).  We have used a related dye, Procion Red HE3B (whose structure
has not been released by the manufacturers), to purify the reductase.  The structures
of two related dyes are shown in Fig. 5.  The use of Procion Red HE3B-Sepharose in
protein purification was originally reported by Baird *et al.* (61) and has since
been used to purify a number of dehydrogenases (62).  Ox brain methylene-FH$_4$ reductase partially purified by DEAE-cellulose chromatography (22) was applied to a
column of Red HE3B-Sepharose equilibrated in 50 mM potassium phosphate buffer, pH
7.0.  After elution of unabsorbed protein, reductase activity was eluted by means
of a linear gradient of KCl (0-3 M) Fig. 6).  The enzyme was purified a further 50-

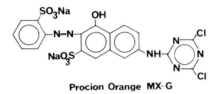

Fig. 5.   The structures of two chlorotriazinyl dyes: Procion Red
H3B and Procion Orange MX-G.

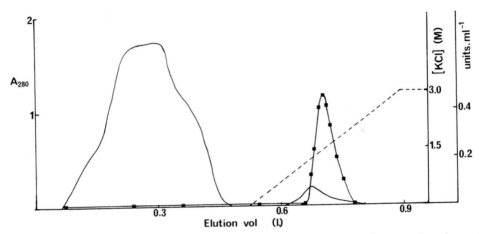

Fig. 6. Purification of ox brain methylene-FH$_4$ reductase by chromatography on Procion Red HE3B-Sepharose. Methylene-FH$_4$ reductase
partially purified by chromatography on DEAE-cellulose was applied to a column of Red-Sepharose equilibrated with 50 mM
potassium phosphate buffer, pH 7.2. The column was washed with
equilibration buffer until A$_{280}$ = 0 and enzyme activity was then
eluted by a linear gradient (0 - 3 M) of KCl. Fractions were
collected and the enzyme activity (■——■) and A$_{280}$ (———) of
the fractions were measured.

fold by this technique and retained the purported dopamine methyltransferase activity as measured by the method of Laduron, providing further evidence for the identity of these two activities.

The sensitivity of the reductase to possible inhibitors is shown in Table 6.   The
enzyme was significantly inhibited by folate analogs, of which the most potent was

trimethoprim.  A number of reports have demonstrated a relationship between the
levels of anticonvulsants and folate derivatives during the treatment of epilepsy.
However of the anticonvulsants tested none significantly affected reductase activity.  The mechanism by which anticonvulsants affect folate levels remains unclear.

TABLE VI.    SENSITIVITY OF METHYLENE-FH$_4$ REDUCTASE TO DRUGS

| Addition | % Activity |
|---|---|
| None | 100 |
| Aminopterin | 70 |
| Methotrexate | 60 |
| Dichloromethotrexate | 55 |
| Trimethoprim | 50 |
| Diphenylhydantoin | 100 |
| Barbitone | 100 |
| Phenobarbitone | 100 |
| Sodium Valproate | 100 |
| Chlorpromazine | 100 |
| Trifluoperazine | 100 |
| Procion Red HE3B | <1 |
| Cibacron Blue F3GA | <1 |

All additives were at a final concentration of 100 µM.  Assays were performed at pH 7.2 using the spectrophotometric method of Kutzbach and Stokstad (Ref. 20).

The postulate that folate-dependent methylation may be promoted in brain in schizophrenia (49) is now obviously untenable, in view of the apparent artefactual nature of this reaction.  However, there are other suggestive links between abnormalities in folate metabolism and mental illness [see Turner (63) for review].  Of principal interest is the report that the levels of methylene-FH4 reductase in brain may be reduced in schizophrenia and that administration of folic acid could reduce the psychotic symptoms (64).  However, neuroleptic drugs (e.g. chlorpromazine and trifluperazine) did not affect the brain methylene-FH$_4$ reductase activity (Table 6). We are currently undertaking a study of the levels of folate-dependent enzymes in post-mortem brain samples from control and schizophrenic patients.

SAM has been reported to regulate the activity of methylene-FH$_4$ reductase in liver and brain (see above and Ref. 20).  In liver, half-maximal inhibition of methylene-FH$_4$ reductase was reported to occur at a concentration of 2.8 µM SAM, which was

raised to 5 µM in the presence of 2 µM SAH.  It seems unlikely that such potent inhibition would occur in brain since reductase activity, and therefore the major pathway to SAM synthesis, would be switched off under normal conditions in this tissue.
Burton and Sallach (23) have reported that 2 mM SAM produced more than 90% inhibition of brain reductase activity, whereas Ordónez and Wurtman (17) have claimed that
physiological concentrations of SAM (0.8 mM) produced only 36% inhibition.  However,
one should bear in mind that the enzyme is easily de-sensitized to inhibition by
procedures such as dialysis at $0^{\circ}C$ (65).  We have therefore examined the effects of
SAM and SAH at millimolar concentrations on the activity of rat brain methylene-$FH_4$
reductase.  A cytosolic extract of brain that had been gel-filtered and assayed immediately was used in order to minimize de-sensitization.  The data presented in
Fig. 7 suggests that the brain reductase is less sensitive to inhibition than that

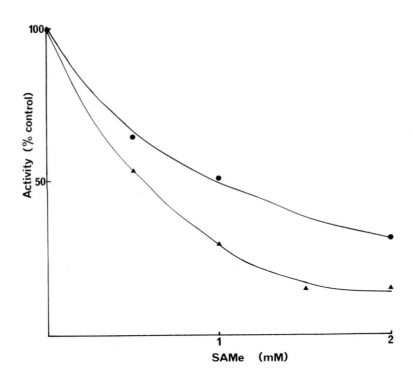

Fig. 7.   Effects of adenosyl methionine (SAM) and adenosyl homocysteine
          (SAH) on the activity of methylene-$FH_4$ reductase from rat brain.
          A freshly prepared cytosolic fraction from rat brain was gel-
          filtered on a column of Sephadex G50 to remove endogenous SAM
          and then assayed radiometrically at $30^{\circ}C$ in the presence of
          various concentrations of SAM (▲——▲) or various concentra-
          tions of SAM together with 1 mM SAH (●——●).  Results are ex-
          pressed at % activity in the absence of SAM.

reported for liver enzyme and the degree of inhibition observed would not be incompatible with a physiological regulation of the brain reductase by SAM.  SAH could partially reverse this inhibition.

## DISCUSSION

The folate-dependent methyl transferase enjoyed a brief and chequered life.  The majority of the activity attributed to this enzyme was shown to be due to the action of methylene-$FH_4$ reductase acting in the reverse of its presumed physiological direction.  The major products of the reaction between $CH_3FH_4$ and biogenic amines have now been characterized as alicyclic alkaloids formed by the non-enzymic condensation of the amines with formaldehyde.  The identity of the products has been confirmed by mass spectroscopy and has provided a cautionary warning about relying on a single method of product identification such as thin-layer chromatography.  However, the ease with which tetrahydroisoquinoline and tryptoline alkaloids can be formed *in vitro* has led to a good deal of speculation about the possible formation of these metabolites *in vivo*.

The production of isoquinoline and β-carboline alkaloids from endogenous amines and acetaldehyde has been implicated in the process of ethanol dependence (67), and the condensation product of acetaldehyde with dopamine (salsolinol) has been identified in the brains of ethanol-intoxicated rats (68).  Such alkaloids have been shown to inhibit the uptake and retention of neurotransmitter amines in synaptosome preparations (69) and to inhibit monoamine oxidase activity (70).  However, convincing evidence for a physiological role of these compounds in brain function remains to be established (see 71 for further discussion).  There is no evidence to date that tryptolines can form *in vivo* as a consequence of the action of methylene-$FH_4$ reductase and it has been a basic tenet of folate research that this enzyme functions physiologically in the direction of $CH_3FH_4$ formation (26).  However this principle may have to be revised as a result of recent studies by Ordonez and Caraballo (58) who have examined the developmental characteristics of methylene-$FH_4$ reductase in brain.  The activity of this enzyme was maximal in neo-natal rats and declined to 20% of this maximal level in adult rats.  Thus it has been suggested that in early stages of development the reductase may play a role in oxidizing $CH_3FH_4$ transported into brain to methylene-$FH_4$, thereby contributing to the one-carbon pool for thymidine biosynthesis (58).  If this observation were to be confirmed, it would be of interest to compare the regulatory characteristics of methylene-$FH_4$ reductase prepared from young and adult rats.  The demonstration in this paper that serine hydroxymethyltransferase can also participate in tryptoline biosynthesis has provided an alternative metabolic route by which these alkaloids may be formed *in vivo* and will hopefully lead to further research into the possible physiological role of these compounds.

The incorrect identification of amine metabolites by thin-layer chromatography has also called into question the identity of the products formed by incubation of tryptamine with SAM and brain extract (38, 39). A proportion of the products formed in this case may also correspond with tryptoline-like alkaloids. Some authors (38) have been unable to detect significant formation in brain of N-methyl tryptamine from tryptamine and SAM, although the activity in lung tissue can easily be measured. It therefore appears that the radiochemical assay previously used for the measurement of indoleamine N-methyl transferase activity in brain may be inadequate and a procedure involving gas chromatography coupled with mass spectroscopy would be preferable wherever possible (39). A recent report using this technique has shown low but detectable activity of SAM-dependent transferase in brain (2-pmol N-methyl tryptamine formed/h/mg protein) (39). Interestingly these authors reported that using a lung extract and $CH_3FH_4$ as methyl donor there was detectable formation of N-methyl tryptamine as identified by mass spectroscopy. The enzyme preparation in this case had been extensively dialyzed so it was unlikely that the reaction involved SAM as an obligatory intermediate. Thus the folate-dependent methylation story may be down but not quite out.

The reports of a possible role of folic acid derivatives in neurotransmitter metabolism has promoted renewed interest in all aspects of the metabolism and functions of folates in brain. Their role in the provision of precursors for nucleic acid metabolism and hence in the maturation of the nervous system is well established. Their role in aspects of transmitter metabolism in the mature brain should provide a fruitful area of research for some years to come, particularly in view of the neurological conditions that have been associated with deficiencies in folate metabolism (63, 72). Studies on the enzymology of folate metabolism have been limited to date by the instability of the substrates and limited availability of the polyglutamate forms of the folates, which in many cases, are the preferred substrates for folate-metabolizing enzymes (73, 74). Furthermore, no folate-enzyme has yet been obtained in a homogenous form from nervous tissue. However, a clearer picture of the relation between folates, SAM and neurotransmitter metabolism is already appearing, although the confusion that has proliferated in this area in recent years leaves the path of the research worker best summarized as follows:

> "Nel mezzo del cammin di nostra vita mi ritrovai per una
> selva oscura che la diritta via era smarrita"
>
> (Dante Alighieri, La Divina Commedia)

ACKNOWLEDGEMENTS

We should like to thank the Medical Research Council for financial support and BioResearch, Milan for a generous supply of SAM.

REFERENCES

1.  Blakley, R.L., The Biochemistry of Folic Acid and Related Pteridines, North-Holland, Amsterdam (1969).

2.  Spector, R., Lorenzo, A.V. and Drug, D.E., Biochem. Pharmac., 24, 542 (1975).

3.  Spector, R. and Lorenzo, A.V., Science, N.Y., 187, 540 (1975).

4.  Korevaar, W.C., Geyer, M.A., Knapp, S., Hsu, L.L. and Mandell, A.J., Nature New Biol., 245, 244 (1973).

5.  Makulu, D.R., Smith, E.F. and Bertino, J.R., J. Neurochem., 21, 241 (1973).

6.  Spector, R., Levy, P. and Abelson, H.T., Biochem. Pharmac., 26, 1507 (1977).

7.  Lynn, R., Reuter, M.E. and Guynn, R.W., J. Neurochem., 29, 1147 (1977).

8.  Pollock, R.J. and Kaufman, S., J. Neurochem., 30, 253 (1978).

9.  Spector, R., Levy, P. and Abelson, H.T., J. Neurochem., 29, 919 (1977).

10. Algeri, S., Bonati, M., Brunello, N. and Ponzio, F., Brain Res., 132, 569 (1977).

11. Craine, J.E., Hall, E.S. and Kaufman, S., J. Biol. Chem., 247, 6082 (1972).

12. Kaufman, B.T. and Gardiner, R.C., J. Biol. Chem., 241, 1319 (1966).

13. Rowe, P.B. and Russell, P.J., J. Biol. Chem., 248, 984 (1973).

14. Turner, A.J., Ponzio, F. and Algeri, S., Brain Res., 70, 553 (1974).

15. Finkelstein, J.D., Kyle, W.E. and Harris, B.J., Arch. Biochem. Biophys., 146, 84 (1971).

16. Langer, B.W., Proc. Soc. Exp. Biol. Med., 115, 1088 (1964).

17. Ordóñez, L.A. and Wurtman, R.J., J. Neurochem., 21, 1447 (1973).

18. McClain, L.D., Carl, G.F. and Bridgers, W.F., J. Neurochem., 24, 719 (1975).

19. Daly, E.C., Nadi, N.S. and Aprison, M.H., J. Neurochem., 26, 179 (1976).

20. Kutzbach, C. and Stokstad, E.L.R., Biochim. Biophys. Acta., 250, 459 (1971).

21. Pearson, A.G.M., Ph.D. thesis, University of Leeds (1978).

22. Pearson, A.G.M. and Turner, A.J., Nature, 258, 173 (1975).

23. Burton, E.G. and Sallach, H.J., Arch. Biochem. Biophys., 166, 483 (1975).

24. Deguchi, T. and Barchas, J., J. Biol. Chem., 246, 3175 (1971).

25.  Walker, R.D. and Duerre, J.A., *Can. J. Biochem.*, 53, 312 (1975).

26.  Herbert, V. and Zalusky, R., *J. Clin. Invest.*, 41, 1263 (1962).

27.  Daly, E.C. and Aprison, M.H., *J. Neurochem.*, 22, 877 (1974).

28.  Rassin, D.K. and Gaull, G.E., *J. Neurochem.*, 24, 969 (1975).

29.  McClain, L.D., Carl, G.F. and Bridgers, W.F., *J. Neurochem.*, 24, 719 (1975).

30.  Davies, L.P. and Johnston, G.A.R., *Brain Res.*, 54, 149 (1973).

31.  Cybulski, R.L. and Fisher, R.R., *Biochem.*, 15, 3183 (1976).

32.  Axelrod, J., *Science*, 134, 343 (1961).

33.  Mandel, L.R., Rosenzweig, S. and Kuehl, F.A., *Biochem. Pharmac.*, 20, 712 (1971).

34.  Mandel, A.J. and Morgan, M., *Nature New Biol.*, 230, 85 (1971).

35.  Saavedra, J.M., Coyle, J.T. and Axelrod, J., *J. Neurochem.*, 20, 743 (1973).

36.  Saavedra, J.M., *Essays Neurochem. Neuropharmac.*, 1, 1 (1977).

37.  Marzullo, G., Rosengarten, H. and Friedhoff, A.J., *Life Sci.*, 20, 775 (1977).

38.  Gomes, U.R., Neethling, A.C. and Shanley, B.C., *J. Neurochem.*, 27, 701 (1976).

39.  Boarder, M.R. and Rodnight, R., *Brain Res.*, 114, 359 (1976).

40.  Mandel, L.R., Prasad, R., Lopez-Ramos, B. and Walker , R.W., *Res. Commun. Chem. Path. Pharmac.*, 16, 47 (1977).

41.  Laduron, P., *Nature New Biol.*, 238, 212 (1972).

42.  Laduron, P., Gommeren, W.R. and Leysen, J.E., *Biochem. Pharmac.*, 23, 1599 (1974).

43.  Cantoni, G.L., in *Comp. Biochem.*, Florkin, M. and Mason, H., Eds., Academic Press, New York, 1, 181 (1960).

44.  Caotoni, G.L., *Ann. Rev. Biochem.*, 44, 435 (1975).

45.  Banerjee, S.P. and Snyder, S.H., *Science*, 182, 74 (1973).

46.  Hsu, L.L. and Mandell, A.J., *Life Sci.*, 13, 847 (1973).

47.  Snyder, S.H., Banerjee, S.P., Yamamura, H.T. and Greenberg, D., *Science*, 184, 1243 (1974).

48.  Kersten, H., Sandig, L. and Arnold, H.H., *FEBS Lett.*, 55, 57 (1975).

49.  Laduron, P., *J. Psychiat. Res.*, 11, 257 (1974).

50.  Lin, R.-L. and Narasimhachari, N., *Res. Commun. Chem. Path. Pharmac.*, 8, 535 (1974).

51.  Mandel, L.R., Rosegay, A., Walker, R.W., Vandenheuval, W.J.A. and Rokach, J., *Science*, 186, 741 (1974).

52. Wyatt, R.J., Erdelyi, E., DoAmaral, J.R., Elliott, G.R., Renson, J and Barchas, J.D., _Science_, 187, 853 (1975).

53. Meller, E., Rosengarten, H., Friedhoff, A.J., Stebbins, R.D. and Silber, R., _Science_, 187, 171 (1975).

54. Ungar, F., Tabakoff, B. and Alivisatos, S.G.A., _Biochem. Pharmac._, 22, 1905 (1973).

55. Uotila, L. and Koivusalo, M., _J. Biol. Chem._, 249, 7653 (1974).

56. Katzen, H.M. and Buchanan, J.M., _J. Biol. Chem._, 240, 825 (1965).

57. Taylor, R.T. and Hanna, M.L., _Life Sci._, 17, 111 (1975).

58. Ordonez, L.A. and Caraballo, F., _Psychopharmac. Commun._, 1, 253 (1975).

59. Jones, C.W. and Priest, D.G., _Arch. Biochem. Biophys._, 174, 305 (1976).

60. Thompson, S.T., Cass, K.H. and Stellwagen, E., _Proc. Nat. Acad. Sci._, USA, 72, 669 (1975).

61. Baird, J.K., Sherwood, R.F., Carr, R.J.G. and Atkinson, A., _FEBS Lett._, 70, 61 (1976).

62. Stockton, J., Pearson, A.G.M., West, L.J. and Turner, A.J., _Biochem. Soc. Trans._, (1978) in press.

63. Turner, A.J., _Biochem. Pharmac._, 26, 1009 (1977).

64. Mudd, S.H. and Freeman, J.M., _J. Psychiat. Res._, 11, 259 (1974).

65. Kutzbach, C. and Stokstad, E.L.R., _Biochim. Biophys. Acta._, 139, 217 (1967).

66. Hsu, L.L. and Mandell, A.J., _J. Neurochem._, 24, 631 (1975).

67. Rahwan, R.G., _Toxicol. Appl. Pharmac._, 34, 3 (1975).

68. Collins, M.A. and Bigdeli, M.G., _Life Sci._, 16, 585 (1975).

69. Alpers, H.S., McLaughlin, B.R., Nix, W.N. and Davis, V.E., _Biochem. Pharmac._, 24, 1391 (1975).

70. Meller, E., Friedman, E., Schweitzer, J.W. and Friedhoff, A.J., _J. Neurochem._, 28, 995 (1977).

71. Tipton, K.F., Houslay, M.D. and Turner, A.J., _Essays Neurochem. Neuropharmac._, 1, 103 (1977).

72. Erbe, R.W., _New Engl. J. Med._, 293, 753 (1975).

73. Blakley, R.L., _Biochem. J._, 65, 342 (1957).

74. Coward, J.K., Parameswaran, K.N., Cashmore, A.R. and Bertino, J.R., _Biochem._, 13, 3899 (1974).

# Dietary Influences on Brain Neurotransmitter Synthesis and Brain Methylation Reactions

**Richard J. Wurtman**

Laboratory of Neuroendocrine Regulation, Massachusetts Institute of Technology, Cambridge, Massachusetts

The brain has long been thought to occupy so exalted a position among the organs of the body that its metabolic needs are invariably the first to be met. Thus, if the quantities of oxygen, glucose, or heat present in the blood were in short supply, the scarce item would preferentially be utilized by the brain. An unstated corollary of this formulation is that, under normal conditions, the amounts of circulating nutrients available to the brain at any moment are largely independent of their concentrations in the blood: the brain knows what substances it requires, and takes them from the circulation, oblivious to the dietary history or metabolic state of its host.

We and our associates at MIT (notably John Fernstrom, Edith Cohen, and Candace Gibson) have been surprised to discover that this view of the brain as an autonomous organ, independent (except perhaps in certain disease states) of metabolic processes elsewhere in the body, is no longer tenable. In fact, the ability of brain neurons to make and release at least two neurotransmitters (serotonin and acetylcholine – and probably the catecholamines) depends directly on the composition of the blood, and consequently on what foods have most recently been consumed.

We have found that each meal can, depending on its composition, alter brain tryptophan and choline levels, and thereby modify the functional activities of neurons that function by releasing serotonin or acetylcholine from their nerve terminals (1,2). As is described below, brain·tryptophan levels depend primarily on the proportions of carbohydrate and protein in the meal, while choline levels depend on the diet's lecithin content. We were initially surprised when we discovered that neurons releasing serotonin were normally susceptible to the vagaries of food choice; we have been all the more astonished to find similar vulnerabilities among cholinergic and catecholaminergic neurons and in the ability of brain cells to synthesize S-adenosyl-methionine (SAM – which, as described below, varies with their concentrations of methionine, its amino acid precursor). We are a long way from understanding why the evolutionary process apparently allowed to arise and persist

71

such "open-loop" control of these important molecules. However, this poverty of
imagination has not deterred a number of laboratories, including our own, both to
learn more about how it functions normally, and to begin to treat disease states
related to the brain constituents that are precursor-dependent (3).

NEUROTRANSMITTERS

All of the known neurotransmitters synthesized in mammalian neurons share certain
chemical properties: all are low molecular weight, water-soluble compounds which
are ionized at pH of body fluids. All are synthesized primarily in the parts of
the neuron (the synaptic bulbs, or nerve terminals) which form synaptic contacts
with the cells to which the neuron transmits signals (the postsynaptic cells), and
all are stored within subcellular organelles (synaptic vesicles) or are attached
to cytoplasmic proteins, prior to being released into a synapse. Release occurs
when the neuron that synthesized the neurotransmitter is depolarized. Thereafter,
some of the transmitter molecules released come into contact with receptors on the
surface of the postsynaptic cell. This interaction ultimately leads to a change in
the rate at which a particular ion (e.g., sodium or chloride) enters the postsynaptic cell; such ionic alterations determine whether or not will occur a depolariza-
tion. A given postsynaptic neuron may be impinged on by neurotransmitters released
from perhaps as many as 10,000 presynaptic neurons. Some of the transmitters (like
acetylcholine) are excitatory, in that the changes in ionic fluxes that they produce enhance the liklihood that the postsynaptic cell will become deploarized.
Others (like serotonin) are inhibitory, causing the potential of the postsynaptic
cell membrane to become less likely to depolarize. At any given instant, the postsynaptic cell membrane summates all of its ionic responses to the excitatory and
inhibitory transmitters that happen to be impinging on it, and somehow determines
whether or not to depolarize.

At the present time, about 15-20 compounds have been identified in mammalian central
nervous systems that probably function as neurotransmitters. We suspect that these
putative transmitters can be classified in one of three groups, depending on their
probable modes of synthesis. As we shall see, only for one of these groups does it
seem likely that the rate of neurotransmitter synthesis might normally be coupled
to plasma composition and food consumption.

Group I includes, in addition to serotonin and acetylcholine, histamine (4) and the
catecholamine transmitters dopamine and norepinephrine (5). Each of these compounds
is synthesized from a precursor that neurons cannot make, and which thus must be obtained from the circulation. The synthesis of each is catalyzed by an enzyme (e.g.,
tryptophan hydroxylase for serotonin; choline acetyltransferase for acetylcholine;
tyrosine hydroxylase for dopamine and norepinephrine) that has a relatively low af-

finity for its substrate, and which thus normally operates at less-than-maximal
efficiency (i.e., because it virtually never is fully saturated with the tryptophan
or choline). Group II includes the various peptides that have been found in brain
neurons and are thought by many scientists to function as neurotransmitters, largely
because of their presence in neurons and their ability to modify ionic fluxes when
applied to brain neurons. These compounds almost certainly are synthesized not by
enzymes but by polyribosomes (i.e., strands of messenger RNA attached to ribosomes).
The concentrations of amino acids needed to allow polysome-directed peptide synthesis to occur at maximal rates in brain apparently are quite low; hence, it doesn't
seem likely that normal, food-induced variations in plasma amino acid levels will
be found to have much effect on the formation of the peptide neurotransmitters.
Group III includes three amino acids that can be synthesized by all cells (glycine,
glutamate, and aspartate), and a fourth amino acid, GABA (gamma-amino butyric acid),
formed in brain neurons from glutamate. Since all neurons are able to synthesize
glycine, glutamate, and aspartate from glucose or any other energy source, it also
seems unlikely that the production of these four neurotransmitters will be found·
to vary normally with food consumption or plasma composition. (However, no data are
available from experiments examining the nutritional control of their synthesis in
brain, and the possibility that they are under such control must still be kept open.)

In order to demonstrate that a particular neurotransmitter falls within Group I, and
is thus subject to nutritional control, it appears that five types of evidence must
be obtained:  A) brain neurons must not be able to synthesize the transmitter's precursor from glucose or any other energy source; B) the brain must be able to obtain
the precursor by taking it up from the circulation; (the uptake system, localized
within the brain capillaries at the site of the blood-brain barrier, should also
exhibit only a low affinity for the precursor, thereby allowing the rate at which
uptake occurs when plasma levels of the precursor rise and fall); C) plasma levels
of the precursor must rise and fall (e.g. in response to eating, or to fasting, or
to the secretion of one or more hormones); D) the key regulatory enzyme that the
neurons use to convert the precursor to the neurotransmitter should also, as described above, have a low affinity for the precursor (and thus normally function at
less-than-maximal efficiency); and no closed feedback loops should operate within
the neuron to keep its neurotransmitter levels constant (e.g., if the concentrations
of the neurotransmitter within the neuron feeds back onto the control enzyme involved in its synthesis, decreasing the enzyme's activity when transmitter concentrations became elevated, then an increase in precursor levels couldn't cause a prolonged acceleration in the synthesis of the neurotransmitter). These criteria, and
the proposed classification of neurotransmitters based on their mode of synthesis,
were arrived at only slowly, as it became established that the synthesis of sero-

tonin, and then of acetylcholine, SAM, and other brain constituents could be normally under precursor control.

SEROTONIN

Our initial studies, started in 1970, were designed to determine whether the increase in brain serotonin levels previously observed in rats given a large dose of
tryptophan (6) might be indicative of changes that <u>normally</u> occur when plasma tryptophan levels rise, such as after eating.  To this end, we first obtained blood and
brain samples from animals sacrificed at various times of day and night, to char-
acterize the normal variations in tryptophan and serotonin.  We found that, immediately after the onset of darkness, when rats normally begin to eat, parallel
elevations occurred in blood and brain tryptophan levels, and soon thereafter, in
brain serotonin concentrations (7).  These findings first suggested that serotonin
synthesis in brain neurons might normally be coupled to plasma tryptophan concentrations, which in turn changed following the ingestion of food.  Further evidence
supporting this hypothetical relationship was obtained by injecting rats with very
small doses of tryptophan, at a time of day (noon) when blood and brain tryptophan
levels are normally lowest, and showing that the increases in brain tryptophan
caused by this treatment also were associated with increases in brain serotonin (1).
In subsequent studies, the injection of insulin, which raises plasma tryptophan
levels in the rat (8), were also observed to cause the now-anticipated rise in
brain tryptophan and serotonin (9).  At this point, we decided to see whether the
secretion of the animal's own insulin similarly affected brain serotonin synthesis.
We fasted rats overnight, then gave them free access for two hours to a carbohydrate
meal which, we knew, would elicit insulin secretion.  To our surprise and delight,
consumption of this single meal caused sequential elevations in blood tryptophan,
brain tryptophan, and brain serotonin levels (9).  Thus was it first shown that
eating, <u>per se</u>, could normally affect the synthesis of a brain neurotransmitter.

If a large amount of protein was added to the meal, the resulting changes in both
brain tryptophan and serotonin were the opposite of what we had originally antici-
pated: both fell.  Protein contains tryptophan, and contributes some of its tryptophan molecules to the blood after its ingestion.  Thus, we assumed that the addition
of protein to the meal would be associated with an increase in brain tryptophan.
The fact that the opposite change occurs was ultimately shown to be realated to the
properties of the system that transports tryptophan across the blood-brain barrier
and into the brain.  This same system also transports numerous other neutral amino
acids found in protein (e.g., tyrosine, methionine, leucine) (10).  When protein is
consumed, the resulting increases in the plasma concentrations of these other amino
acids are greater, proportionately, than that of tryptophan.  Hence, the more protein
in the meal, the lower the ratio in blood of the tryptophan concentration to that of

its neutral amino acid competitors, and thus the slower the uptake of tryptophan into the brain (11). Serotonin-containing neurons thus appear to be variable-ratio sensors, modifying the production, and probably the release, of their neurotransmitter as an inverse function of each meal's protein content. These neurons probably function to provide the brain with information about the peripheral metabolic state, which the brain can use to decide what and when to eat, whether to sleep, when to cause the secretion of particular hormones, and so forth. Changes in most of these and other brain functions have now been observed following the administration of tryptophan or the consumption of meals that modify brain serotonin. The effects of the diet on plasma amino acid levels (and thus, in all likelihood,synthesis), in humans appears to be virtually identical with those observed in the rat.

ACETYLCHOLINE

About four years ago, we began to explore the relationahip between blood choline levels and the synthesis of the neurotransmitter acetylcholine. The enzyme that converts choline to acetylcholine, choline acetyltransferase, was already known to share with tryptophan hydroxylase the property of having a low affinity for its substrate; and thus it probably also was not working at full efficiency at the choline concentrations normally present in the tissues. Hence, it seemed possible that the synthesis of acetylcholine, like that of serotonin, might be accelerated by treatments that increased the levels of its precursor in the brain. To our knowledge, no one had ever previously examined the effects on brain acetylcholine of administering choline to animals. This lacuna probably reflected the great difficulty scientists previously had in examining the effects of any treatment on brain acetylcholine levels: within a few seconds of death, a major fraction of the acetylcholine in the rat brain is destroyed by a ubiquitous enzyme, acetylcholinesterase. Hence, even a 25% increase or decrease in brain acetylcholine concentrations (a rather sizeable change for a neurotransmitter pool) generally might not have been observable when the brain was examined after death. Our first task was to develop a method for circumventing the post-mortem hydrolysis of brain acetylcholine; this was accomplished by killing the animal with a focussed beam of microwave radiation. This treatment simultaneously coagulates all brain proteins, thereby inactivating acetylcholinesterase (and other brain enzymes).

In short order, we found that the administration of choline, by injection or as a constituent of the diet, caused major sequential elevations in serum choline, brain choline, and brain acetylcholine levels (2). Concentrations of the neurotransmitter could be shown to rise within all cholinergic neurons, inside and outside of the brain, and in the portion of the neuron (the nerve terminals) from which it is released into synapses. Subsequent studies have shown that blood choline levels in

humans and experimental animals normally vary as a function of dietary choline content (12); that the effects of dietary choline provided as lecithin (the form in
which it is usually ingested) are, if anything, far greater than those observed
when choline itself is administered (13); that the acetylcholine-forming enzyme is
not subject to end-product feedback control (unpublished observations); and that
increases in acetylcholine levels are, in fact, associated with parallel changes in
the amounts of the transmitter that are released into synapses to act on postsynaptic receptors (14). Exploration of this latter relationship has been facilitated
by the accessibility of the cholinergic nerves located outside of the brain (e.g.,
those that innervate the adrenal medulla and cause it to secrete epiniphrine).

Within four months of the publication of our first article showing that choline administration elevates brain acetylcholine levels in rats, the first note appeared in
a medical journal suggesting a clinical use for this effect. A letter to the editor
of the New England Journal of Medicine by a group of psychiatrists working at Stan-
ford University (15) described marked improvements after choline administration in
a patient suffering from a neurological disease, tardive dyskinesia. (This disease
causes uncontrolled movements of the tongue, mouth, face, and upper trunk; it is a
common side effect associated with the use of all presently-marketed antipsychotic
drugs. In some patients, it may continue indefinitely, long after treatment with
the antipsychotic drug has been discontinued. Similar movement disorders may also
occur spontaneously in patients with no history of having taken antipsychotic drugs.)
On the basis of largely indirect evidence, neurologists and psychiatrists had spec-
ulated for several years that this movement disorder resulted from the release of
inadequate amounts of acetylcholine within the brain. However, no orally effective
compound was available that could be administered chronically to restore normal
cholinergic tone within the brain.

During the past year, choline has been affirmed as a useful therapy for tardive
dyskinesia in a controlled, double-blind, crossover study (3). Twenty patients suffering from chronic tardive dyskinesia received choline or a placebo for two weeks
each. Nine of the patients showed major improvement after choline; none showed any
response to the placebo. No other potentially useful treatment, to our knowledge,
has ever been shown in a controlled study to benefit patients with this disease. In
preliminary studies, we now find that oral choline continues to be effective when
given for long periods, and that lecithin, the natural dietary source of choline, is
probably even more useful than choline itself (since it suppresses the signs of the
disease without causing choline's one overt side-effect, i.e., a fishy odor associated with a compound formed from choline by gut bacteria, trimethylamine). Even
though choline administration apparently suppresses a major side-effect of anti-

psychotic drugs (e.g., tardive dyskinesia), we find no evidence that its administration in any way interferes with the therapeutic actions of these drugs.  This
dissociation may have important implications in helping us to identify the brain
loci involved in causing psychoses.

Similar studies are now underway at M.I.T. and numerous other institutions on the
possible uses of choline or lecithin to treat other diseases that are thought to
involve cholinergic neurons.  These include both brain diseases, such as mania and
memory loss, and peripheral disorders, like the myasthenic syndromes.  The ability
of choline to enhance cholinergic transmission has also proven very useful in basic
science studies designed to explore the functions of cholinergic neurons in the
brain (16).

CATECHOLAMINES

The production and release of the catecholamine neurotransmitters dopamine and norepinephrine can also be influenced by physiologic variations in brain tyrosine levels.
The rate at which brain neurons accumulate dopa after pharmacological inhibition of
dopa decarboxylase - an index of the rate at which they would otherwise synthesize
dopamine or norepinephrine - has been shown to increase when brain tyrosine levels
are elevated (by giving rats tyrosine) and to decrease when tyrosine levels are
lowered (by giving animals a competing neutral amino acid) (5).  The consumption of
individual meals that change brain tyrosine levels also causes the now-expected
changes in brain dopa accumulation: a meal that is relatively rich in protein causes disproportionate increases in plasma tyrosine (because some of the phenylala-
nine in the protein is converted to tyrosine in the liver), thereby increasing both
brain tyrosine levels and the rate of catechol synthesis.  Available evidence suggests that there are some differences between dopaminergic and noradrenergic brain
neurons in the extent to which production of their neurotransmitters depends on
precursor (tryosine) levels: In dopaminergic neurons, the tyrosine hydroxylase must
be activated (e.g., by treating animals with a drug, haloperidol, that accelerates
the neurons' firing rates) in order for tyrosine levels to control dopamine formation (17).  In contrast, in all situations thus far examined,brain norepinephrine
synthesis appears to be precursor-dependent (18).  Precursor-induced changes in
catecholamine synthesis are associated with parallel changes in the release of
dopamine and norepinephrine (as indicated by changes in brain levels of homovanillic
acid and MOPEG sulphate, their major metabolites) (17, 18).

The ability of brain tyrosine levels to affect catecholamine synthesis could have
an even greater impact on clinical problems than the uses described above for choline's effects on acetylcholine.  Norepinephrine-containing neurons are involved in
a very large number of physiological mechanisms, both inside and outside of the

brain, and dopaminergic neurons have clearly been implicated in the etiology of Parkinson's disease. schizophreñia, and other brain disorders.

## S-ADENOSYLMETHIONINE

The synthesis of SAM, like that of the neurotransmitters described above, also is dependent on brain levels of its immediate precursor, methionine: if this amino acid is elevated, either by giving a rat an injection of methionine (19, 20) or by allowing it to consume a single meal that causes an increase in the ratio of plasma methionine levels to those of the competing neutral amino acids (20), sequential elevations are observed in brain methionine and in brain SAM. That exogenous methionine - by changing blood methionine levels - should be able to affect SAM synthesis is perhaps surprising, inasmuch as the brain is capable of synthesizing methionine by the re-methylation of homocysteine (21). Perhaps circulating methionine is preferentially utilized for SAM synthesis. The other criteria for precursor control apparently are met by methionine-SAM, i.e., blood methionine levels do change post-prandially; the uptake of methionine into the brain is catalyzed by a low-affinity (and hence unsaturated) transport system (i.e., the same system as that responsible for taking up circulating tyrosine and tryptophan) (10); the SAM-forming enzyme has a high $K_m$ for methionine relative to tissue methionine concentrations (22); and this enzyme apparently is not inhibited to any significant extent by local SAM concentrations.

Brain methionine levels can be reduced - and the synthesis and levels of brain SAM decreased, as a result - either by suppressing methionine uptake across the blood-brain barrier or by interfering with the re-methylation of brain homocysteine. The former can be accomplished by giving a rat a large dose of a competing neutral a-mino acid, the latter by making the animal deficient in folic acid (a cofactor used by an enzyme in the re-methylation sequence). Precursor-induced changes in brain SAM levels can significantly affect the brain's ability to methylate various substrates, especially when it is confronted with unusually large quantities of methyl acceptors (e.g., in Parkinsonian patients given the catechol amino acid L-dopa (21).)

## SUMMARY

The rates of synthesis of the neurotransmitters serotonin, acetylcholine, and probably also norepinephrine depend physiologically on the availability to the brain of their precursor molecules, tryptophan, choline and tyrosine, respectively. The brain concentration of each precursor can rapidly be influenced by the diet; food ingestion thus readily modifies the syntheses of each of these neurotransmitters in brain. Brain neurons that utilize serotonin, acetylcholine, or norepinephrine are involved in neuronal networks that control a number of body functions and behaviors.

Dietary manipulations (or the consumption of individual nutrients) can thus be used in the therapy of certain brain diseases and in the experimental analysis of functions mediated by monoaminergic or cholinergic neurons.

The synthesis of SAM from the amino acid methionine is also precursor-dependent; brain SAM levels increasing rapidly after rats receive methionine or ingest a high-protein meal that increases brain methionine levels. The brain obtains part of its methionine from the circulation (and, ultimately, from the diet); it also is capable of regulating methionine by re-methylating homocysteine. Brain methionine levels can be decreased by interfering with the availability of either source (e.g., by giving animals large doses of an amino acid that competes with methionine for brain uptake, or by causing folic acid deficiency – which interferes with the methylation of homocysteine). The consequent reductions in SAM synthesis can interfere with the brain's ability to methylate neurotransmitters and other compounds, especially when confronted with unusually large amounts of methyl receptors (e.g., in patients receiving the catechol amino acid L-dopa).

## ACKNOWLEDGEMENTS

The studies described in this report have been supported by grants from the John A. Hartford Foundation, the Ford Foundation, the National Aeronautics and Space Administration, and the United States Public Health Service.

## REFERENCES

1.  Fernstrom, J.D. and Wurtman, R.J., Science, 173, 149 (1971).

2.  Cohen, E.L. and Wurtman, R.J., Science, 16, 1095 (1975).

3.  Growdon, J.H., Hirsch, M.J., Wurtman, R.J. and Weiner, W., New England J. Med., 297, 524 (1977).

4.  Schwartz, J.C., Lampart, C. and Rose, C., J. Neurochem., 19, 801 (1972).

5.  Wurtman, R.J., Larin, F., Mostafapour, S. and Fernstrom, J.D., Science, 185, 183 (1974).

6.  Moir, A.T.B. and Eccleston, D., J. Neurochem., 15, 1093 (1968).

7.  Wurtman, R.J. and Fernstrom, J.D., in Perspectives in Neuropharmacology, Snyder, S.H., Ed., Oxford University Press, New York, 143 (1972).

8.  Fernstrom, J.D. and Wurtman, R.J., Metabolism, 21, 337 (1972).

9.  Fernstrom, J.D. and Wurtman, R.J., Science, 174, 1023 (1971).

10. Pardridge, W.M., in Nutrition and the Brain, R. J. Wurtman and J.J. Wurtman, Eds., Raven Press, New York, 141 (1977).

11. Fernstrom, J.D. and Wurtman, R.J., Science, 178, 414 (1972).

12. Cohen, E.L. and Wurtman, R.J., Science, 191, 561 (1976).

13. Hirsch, M.J. and Wurtman, R.J., Federation Proceedings, 37, 819 (1977).

14. Ulus, I., Hirsch, M.J. and Wurtman, R.J., Proc. Nat. Acad. Sci., 74, 798 (1977).

15. Davis, K.L., Berger, P.A., and Hollister, L.E., New. Eng. J.Med., 293, 152 (1975).

16. Botticelli, L.J., Lytle, L.D. and Wurtman, R.J., Communications in Psychopharm., 1, 519 (1977).

17. Scally, M.J. and Wurtman, R.J., J. Neural Trans., 41, 1 (1977).

18. Gibson, C.J. and Wurtman, R.J., Life Sciences, in press. (1978).

19. Baldessarini, R.J. and Kopin, I.J., J. Neurochem., 13, 769 (1966).

20. Rubin, R.A., Ordonez, L.A. and Wurtman, R.J., J. Neurochem., 23, 227 (1974)

21. Ordonez, L.A. and Wurtman, R.J., Arch. Biochem. Biophys., 160, 372 (1974).

22. Pan, F. and Tarver, H., Arch. Biochem. Biophys., 119, 429 (1967)

# Changes in Rat Brain Noradrenaline and Serotonin Metabolism after Administration of S-Adenosylmethionine

**Sergio Algeri, Emilia Catto, Maria Curcio, Franca Ponzio and Giorgio Stramentinoli**

Istituto di Richerche Farmacologiche, "Mario Negri", Via Eritrea, 62
20157 Milano, Italia

Several authors have reported that S-adenosylmethionine (SAM) shows psychoactive properties when administered to some psychiatric patients (1, 2). As SAM is involved in numerous metabolic pathways (3) in the living organism, it is likely that exogenous SAM may also affect such processes. In view of the possible relationship between affective disorders and central monoaminergic system dysfunction (4), we have directed our attention to the effects of SAM on the metabolism of biogenic amines. 0-Methylation of catecholamines is one of the ways by which these neurotransmitters are inactivated. Transmethylating reactions also occur in the biosynthetic pathways of epinephrine from norepinephrine (NE) and melatonin from serotonin (5-HT). The results presented here, however, show that SAM administration to Sprague-Dawley rats (150-200 g) affects NE and 5-HT metabolism in a completely unexpected way. Effects on the dopaminergic system have so far been less evident, and as research on this aspect is still in progress it will not be discussed in this presentation.

## CHANGES IN NOREPINEPHRINE METABOLISM AFTER SAM ADMINISTRATION

In the experiment described in Fig. 1, SAM was injected three times (50 + 50 i.m. + 100 mg i.v./kg) at 12-h intervals, and the rats were killed 1 h after the last injection. NE levels were determined (5) in an area rich in noradrenergic cell bodies (lower brainstem) and in the hypothalamus, which is rich in noradrenergic nerve terminals. A rapid and pronounced increase of this monoamine (60 and 90%) followed by a slow decline to normal levels was seen in both regions.

As the functional meaning of an increase of neurotransmitter concentration is ambiguous, this preliminary experiment was followed by a study of the effect of SAM on NE synthesis; we measured the transformation of tyrosine into NE after intraventricular injection of a tracer dose of [$^3$H] L-tyrosine, according to the conversion index (C.I.) proposed by Sedval et al. (6, 7).

$$C.I. = \frac{NE \ dpm/g}{Tyrosine \ sp.act.}$$

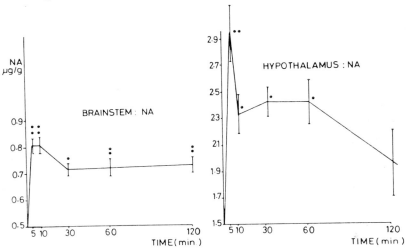

Fig. 1.  NE levels in rat brainstem and hypothalamus at different times
after SAM treatment.  SAM was administered three times (50+50
mg/kg i.m. + 100 mg/kg i.v.) at 12 h intervals.  Rats were killed at different times after the last injection.  Each point is
the mean ± S.E. of 6 determinations.
Statistical significance was analyzed by Duncan's test
● different from control        $p < 0.05$
●● different from control       $p < 0.01$

This study was made in the rat cerebral cortex, an area rich in noradrenergic nerve
terminals.  The animals were treated with SAM as previously indicated.  The results
are summarized in Table 1.  The increase in NE concentration after treatment was

TABLE I.   CORTICAL NOREPINEPHRINE (NE) TURNOVER IN RATS RECEIVING
           S-ADENOSYLMETHIONINE

SAM was administered three times (50 + 50 mg/kg i.m. + 100 mg/kg i.v.) at 12 h interval.  Animals were killed 10 min after intraventricular administration of [3,5-
$^3$H]-L-tyrosine (14 Ci/animal). Data are presented as mean ± S.E. of seven determinations, each made on a pool of three samples.  Statistical significance was analyzed by Student's test.

| Treatment | NE | | C.I. [+++] nmol/g | Tyr. | |
| mg/kg | nmol/g | dpm/nmol | | nmol/g | dpm/nmol |
|---|---|---|---|---|---|
| Vehicle | 1.5±0.03 | 1300±170 | 0.08±0.009 | 123±2.7 | 21300±1300 |
| SAM (50+50+100) | 1.9±0.06 | 1200±120 | 0.16±.022 | 123±4.5 | 18100±2400 |

| SAM I | SAM II | SAM III | $^3$H-Tyr. | Sacr. |
|---|---|---|---|---|
| 12 hr | 12 hr | 1 hr | 10 min | |

+ $p < 0.05$
++ $p < 0.005$
+++ (1) C.I. = Conversion Index = $\dfrac{\text{NE dpm/g tissue}}{\text{Tyr Specific activity}}$

evident in this area too but what is more interesting is that the C.I. is doubled, indicating that NE synthesis was considerably stimulated in these rats.  In this experiment the accumulation of 3-methoxy-4-hydroxyphenylglycol sulfate (MHPG-SO$_4$), the main NE catabolite, was measured in the cerebral cortex of rats treated with SAM (100 mg/kg i/p.) after its egress from the brain had been inhibited by probene- cid treatment (400 mg/kg i.p.). (Fig. 2).  Rats given SAM accumulated the catabolite

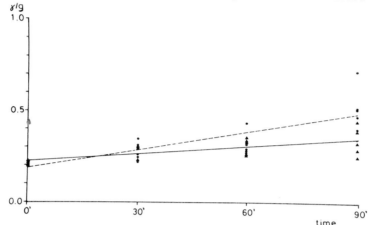

Fig. 2.    Effect of SAM on MHPG-SO$_4$ accumulation in rat cortex after pro-
          benecid administration.
          SAM (100 mg/kg i.p.) was given 5 min before probenecid
          (400 mg/kg i.p.).
          (———▲———) vehicle treated rats  b$_1$  0.00149+0.00067
          (---●---) SAM vehicle treated rats b$_2$ 0.00340+0.00101
          p < 0.05 within confidence limits

at a significantly higher rate than rats given the vehicle only, indicating that treatment with the cofactor stimulates NE turnover.  The fact that in the same an- imals accumulation of HVA, the O-methylated catabolite of DA, was not significantly enhanced (data not presented here) excludes the possibility that the increased MHPG-SO$_4$ formation was due simply to stimulation of the methyl transferase pathway. It is interesting to note that treatment with an equimolecular dose of methionine does not increase MHPG-SO$_4$ formation (Fig. 3).  This is in agreement with the fact that treatment with SAM precursor, i.e., methionine, is not very effective in in- creasing endogenous levels of SAM (8).

## CHANGES IN SEROTONIN METABOLISM AFTER SAM ADMINISTRATION

In another series of experiments we focused our attention on the effect of SAM on 5-HT, another monoamine which appears to be involved in human depression (9).

In the first experiments, rats were treated three times (50 + 50 i.m. + 100 mg i.v./ kg) at 12-h intervals.  5-HT and its catabolite 5-hydroxy indoleacetic acid (5-HIAA) were assayed (10) 1 h after the last injection.  A significant increase in 5-HT and

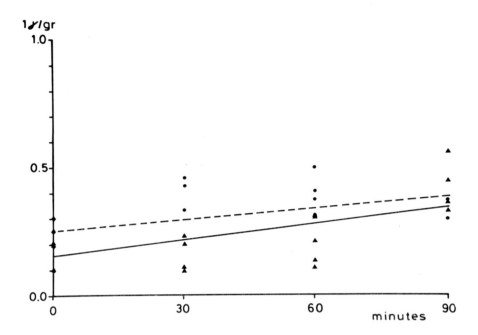

Fig. 3.   Effect of methionine on MHPG-SO$_4$ accumulation in rat cortex after probenecid.   Treatment as in Fig. 2.Methionine was administered in doses equimolecular to 100 mg of SAM (37.5 mg/kg)

5-HIAA was evident in the forebrain, where most of the serotonergic nerve terminals are located (Fig. 4).   In brainstem, an area rich in cell bodies, 5-HIAA levels tended to be higher in SAM-treated animals without reaching statistical significance

In a different experiment, SAM (100 mg/kg) was injected (i.m.) 10 min before and 30 min after an i.v. injection of reserpine (1.25 mg/kg) which depletes brain 5-HT while it increases 5-HIAA formation by impairing the storage mechanism of this monoamine in neuronal granules and making it more available to oxidative enzymes.   Concomitant treatment with SAM did not modify reserpine-depleting action but was able to enhance 5-HIAA formation, suggesting a stimulation of 5-HT synthesis (Fig. 5). This stimulating action of SAM on forebrain 5-HT was confirmed in an experiment in which the rate of 5-HT synthesis after SAM injection (100 + 100 i.m. + 200 mg/kg i.v.) was measured.

Serotonin synthesis was determined by calculating the rates of 5-HT accumulation and 5-HIAA decline after monoamine oxidase inhibition (11).   The results, reported in Fig. 6, show that both 5-HT accumulation and 5-HIAA decline were enhanced in SAM-treated rats, indicating a stimulation of 5-HT turnover.

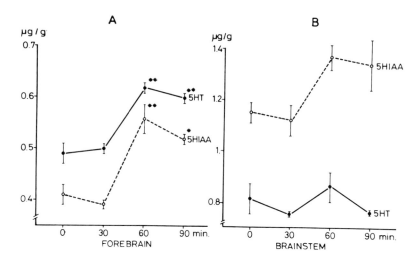

Fig. 4.    Concentration of 5-HT and 5-HIAA in forebrain (A) and brain-
           stem (B) of rats receiving repeated administration of SAM.
           SAM was injected 3 times at 12 h intervals (50 mg + 50 mg/kg
           i.m. + 100 mg/kg i.v.) and the rats were killed 60 min after
           the last injection.
           Seven animals were used for each point.  The results are ex-
           pressed as μg/g of tissue wet weight ± S.E.
           Significance against 0 time group was determined by Duncan's
           new multiple test.

           + p < 0.01
          ++ p < 0.001

Calculation of the turnover rate based on the K of the regression lines gave a value
of 0.24 μg/g/h in the SAM-treated group against 0.14 μg/g/h for controls.  In a dup-
licate experiment the values were 0.19 and 0.13 μg/g/h (12).  The mechanism of action of SAM on brain 5-HT is still unknown.

Serotonin synthesis has been reported to be stimulated by melatonin (13).  In view
of the role of SAM in melatonin biosynthesis and the fact that SAM administration
induced the melatonin-forming enzyme (Stramentinoli, unpublished results), it is
tempting to speculate that this cofactor might indirectly stimulate 5-HT synthesis
through increased melatonin formation.  Work is in progress to test this hypothesis
but other possible mechanisms, such as the formation of some methylated compounds
with psychotropic action (14) or an effect on the formation of some key protein (15),
must also be considered.

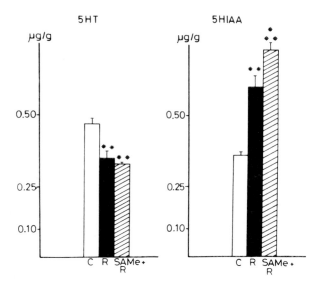

Fig. 5. Interaction of SAM administration with the effect of reserpine on brain 5-HT. Rats were treated with reserpine (R) (1.25 mg/kg i.v.) and SAM vehicle (dark bars) or with SAM (100 mg/kg i.m.) 10 min before and 30 min after injection of reserpine (SAM + R) (hatched bars). Control animals (C) (white bars) received the vehicles only. The animals were killed 70 min after reserpine administration. Each group is the average $\pm$ S.E. of 7 rats.
+ different from R p$<$0.01
++   "   "   " controls p$<$0.01
With Duncan's new multiple test.

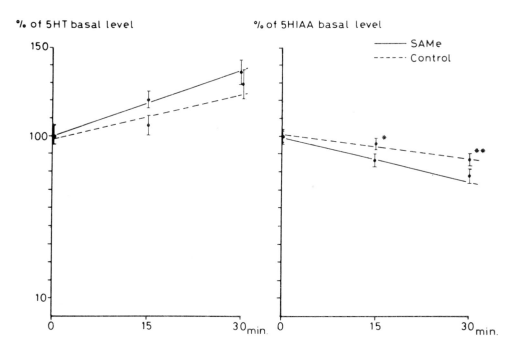

Fig. 6. Rats receiving SAM or its vehicle at 12-h intervals were treated with pargyline (75 mg/kg i.p.) 60 min after the last administration. Turnover rate was calculated by multiplying basal 5-HIAA concentration for the K calculated from the regression lines of 5-HIAA decline. Controls has been determined on the absolute values (13) by a Duncan's new multiple range test.
+  p $<$ 0.05            ++  p $<$ 0.01

CONCLUSION

The experiment presented here indicates that an increase in NE and 5-HT turnover follow the administration of SAM. Although the mechanism of such action is still obscure, these findings show that SAM may affect the metabolism of chemical neurotransmitters in the central nervous system.

REFERENCES

1.  Agnoli, A., Andreoli, V., Casacchia, M. and Cerbo, R., J. Psychiatr. Res., 13, 43 (1976).

2.  Kemali, D., Del Vecchio, M., Vacca, L., Amati, A., Famiglietti, L.A., and Celani, T., this volume.

3.  Cantoni, G.L. in The Biochemistry of Adenosylmethionine, F. Salvatore, E. Borek, V. Zappia, H.G. Willaims-Ashman and F. Schlenk, Eds., Columbia University Press, New York, 557 (1977).

4.  Schildkraut, J.J., Ann. Rev. Pharmacol., 13, 427 (1973).

5.  Chang, C.C., Int. J.Neuropharmacol., 3, 643 (1964).

6.  Sedvall, G.C., Weise, V.K., and Kopin, I.J., J. Pharmacol. Exp. Ther., 159, 274 (1968).

7.  Meek, J.L. and Neff, N.H., Br. J.Pharmacol., 45, 435 (1972).

8.  Stramentinoli, G., Catto, E. and Algeri, S., Commun. Psychopharmacol., 1, 89 (1977).

9.  Asberg, M., Thoren, P., Traskman, L., Bertilsson, L. and Ringberger, V., Science 191, 478 (1976).

10. Curzon, G. and Green, A.R., Br. J. Pharmacol., 39, 653 (1970).

11. Tozer, T.N., Neff, N.H. and Brodie, B.B., J. Pharmacol. Exp. Ther., 153, 177 (1966).

12. Curcio, M., Catto, E., Stramentinoli, G. and Algeri, S., Prog. Neuro-Psychopharmacol., 2, 65 (1978).

13. Anton-Tay, F., Chou, C., Anton, S. and Wurtman, R.J., Science, 162, 277 (1968).

14. Baldessarini, R.J., in Amines and Schizophrenia, H.E. Hemwich, S.S. Kety and J.R. Smythies, Eds., Pergamon Press, Oxford, 199 (1967).

15. Mays, L.L., Borek, E. and Finch, C.E., Nature, 243, 411 (1973).

# Cerebral Utilization of Adenosylmethionine and Adenosylhomocysteine: Effects of Methionine Sulfoximine

**O. Z. Sellinger and R. A. Schatz**

Laboratory of Neurochemistry, Mental Health Research Institute, University of Michigan Medical Center, Ann Arbor, Michigan 48109, USA

The significance of methylation in neural tissue, i.e., the possible special role of the transfer of the methyl group from SAM to neural acceptors with the concomitant formation of SAH, was last reviewed in 1975 (1). Subsequently, two related reviews have appeared, one dealing with the biosynthesis and excretion of hallucinogens formed by methylation of neurotransmitters and related substances (2) and the other reporting on cerebral methionine requirements (3). The possible relationship between methylation and neural excitation first attracted our attention when we noted that SAM levels decreased markedly and regionally in the brain of rats injected with convulsant doses of L-methionine-dl-sulfoximine (4). Since the preconvulsant period after the administration of this agent is sufficiently long (5-6 hours) (5,6) to permit studies of the neurochemical changes associated with and/or responsible for the ensuing seizures (7), we began to examine these changes as they related to methylation in the brain. We have shown elsewhere (8) that the methylation of heterologous transfer ribonucleic acids (tRNAs) by tRNA methyltransferases derived from brains of methionine sulfoximine-pretreated rats is significantly altered, in that methylation of tRNA guanine residues is specifically increased. In the present report we wish to describe the results of our recent work dealing with histamine methylation in the normal and preconvulsant brain and with the modulation of the activity of a partially purified preparation of cerebral histamine N-methyltransferase by several biogenic and methylated "trace" amines. In addition, we also describe some properties of a highly purified preparation of rat brain SAH hydrolase, the enzyme which assures the normal removal from cellular methylation pools of the foremost inhibitor of methylation, SAH.

THE METHYLATION OF HISTAMINE

To explain the observation of decreased SAM levels after methionine sulfoximine we first examined whether this agent blocked the synthesis of SAM. Since this proved

not to be the case (9), we suggested that the administration of methionine sulfoximine somehow resulted in an increased utilization of cerebral SAM, i.e., in an
activation of several of the many methyl transfer reactions taking place in this
organ (10). The choice of the methylation of histamine as one of the methylating
systems of brain with which to test the validity of this suggestion was prompted by
a) The relatively straightforward catabolism of histamine in brain tissue, which
consists of a methylation step to produce a single methylated metabolite, 3-methyl-
histamine, and the further oxidation of the latter to 3-methylimidazoleacetic acid
(11); b) the strict specificity of the histamine methylating enzyme, histamine N-
methyltransferase (12); and c) the emergence of histamine as a possible modulator
of certain expressions of neural activity (13,14).

Initially, we demonstrated that the activity of histamine N-methyltransferase, when
measured in vitro under optimal conditions of substrate saturation, was significantly higher in brains of methionine sulfoximine-treated rats and mice than in corresponding controls (10). We also showed that this effect of methionine sulfoximine
could not be influenced by the administration of a 5:1 molar excess of L-methionine
or by massive doses of L-histidine, suggesting its relative independence of the pre-
vailing brain levels of SAM and of histamine, two substances rapidly formed in brain
from their precursors (15,16). Further, since exhaustive dialysis of homogenates
derived from brains of treated animals prevented the detection of the elevation in
histamine N-methyltransferase, a direct action of methionine sulfoximine "elicits
the accumulation within selected brain cells of methylated, histamine N-methyltrans-
ferase-stimulating substances" (10). To begin testing this notion, we decided to
examine first the effectiveness of several naturally occurring and biologically
potent methylated indoleamines as modulators of histamine N-methyltransferase in
vitro (17). To ensure a high specificity of interaction between the methylated indoleamine ligands and the histamine N-methyltransferase protein, we purified the
enzyme according to the procedure shown in Table 1. More recently, we have replaced
the Sephadex G-100 step with a Sephacryl-200 step followed by a final passage
through a spheroidal hydroxylapatite column. The resulting preparation showed 3
major protein bands on 7.5% polyacrylamine gels (tris-glycine buffer, pH 8.3), only
one of which possessed histamine N-methyltransferase activity, as determined by
direct assay of the extruded band. Elution and re-electrophoresis of the active
band yielded a single, enzymatically active band, as shown in Fig. 1. Tables 2 and
3 illustrate the effect of a number of amines of biological interest on the purified
brain histamine N-methyltransferase, while Fig. 2 depicts the biphasic effect of
variously substituted methyltryptamines, tested over a $10^{-5}M$ - $10^{-8}M$ range and at
$1 \times 10^{-5}M$ (optimal) and $1.25 \times 10^{-6}M$ histamine, on the rat brain enzyme. As pointed out recently (17), these findings reveal that the modulating amines "can go from

TABLE I.   PURIFICATION OF MOUSE BRAIN HISTAMINE N-METHYLTRANSFERASE

| Fraction | Volume (ml) | Protein mg/ml | Protein mg | Total+ activity | Specific++ activity | Purification (x-fold) | Yield (%) |
|---|---|---|---|---|---|---|---|
| Homogenate | 73 | 13.3 | 967 | $1.53 \times 10^6$ | 1,580 | – | 100 |
| 80,000 x g supernatant | 70 | 3.54 | 248 | $7.94 \times 10^5$ | 2,850 | 1.8 | 46.0 |
| Ammonium sulfate ppt. (45–80%) | 10.3 | 2.23 | 22.3 | $8.75 \times 10^5$ | 39,300 | 25.0 | 57.0 |
| DEAE-cellulose | 5.6 | 0.35 | 1.97 | $3.41 \times 10^5$ | 173,320 | 109.2 | 22.0 |
| Sephadex G-100 | 26.3 | 0.034 | 0.93 | $2.47 \times 10^5$ | 261,800 | 166.0 | 16.2 |

+:   dpm $^{14}$[C]-3-methylhistamine/30 min. (8,850 dpm = 1 nmole).

++:  Total activity/total protein.   From (17).

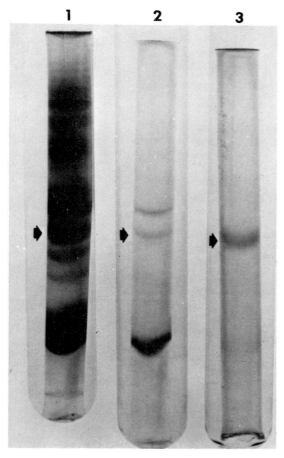

Fig. 1.  Polyacrylamide gel electrophoresis of histamine N-methyltransferase from mouse brain. The gels were 7.5% in polyacrylamide and they were run in 0.39 M tris-glycine buffer, pH 8.3 at 5 mA/gel for approximately 60 minutes. They were stained with Coomassie Blue for 90 minutes and were then electrophoretically destained (P.A.G. Destainer, Shandon Southern) for another 90 minutes. 1) Enzyme after Sephacryl-200, 2) enzyme after hydroxylapatite; 3) the band migrating to the position indicated with arrow in 1 and 2 and which had histamine N-methyltransferase activity, was eluted from II concurrently run gels and the protein eluted by overnight shaking at 4°C in 0.038 M tris-glycine buffer, pH 8.3, containing 1 mM dithiothreitol. The eluted material had enzyme activity and when re-electrophoresed under the conditions specified above it yielded the single band shown, which was enzymatically active, when incubated with histamine and $^{14}$[C]-SAM under the conditions of the histamine N-methyltransferase assay (17).

TABLE II.　THE EFFECT OF AMINES ON RAT AND MOUSE HISTAMINE N-METHYLTRANSFERASE*

| Amine (M) | Rat (2.5 x $10^{-6}$) | Mouse | Rat (1 x $10^{-6}$) | Mouse | Rat (4 x $10^{-7}$) | Mouse |
|---|---|---|---|---|---|---|
| None | 100 | 100 | 100 | 100 | 100 | 100 |
| Tyramine | – | 10 | – | – | – | – |
| Dopamine | 10 | 10 | 18 | 17 | 36 | 30 |
| Octopamine | 45 | – | 64 | – | 82 | – |
| 3-methoxydopamine | 26 | 57 | 37 | 89 | 54 | 96 |
| 4-methoxydopamine | 60 | – | 74 | – | 87 | – |
| Synephrine | 100 | – | 110 | – | 98 | – |
| N-methyldopamine | 85 | – | 88 | – | 93 | – |
| 3,4-dimethoxyphenylethylamine | 85 | – | 99 | – | 94 | – |
| 4-methoxyphenylethylamine | 43 | – | 55 | – | 70 | – |
| Tryptamine | – | – | – | – | – | 35+ |
| 5-hydroxytryptamine | – | 45 | – | – | – | – |
| N-methyltryptamine | 70 | – | 87 | – | 103 | – |
| N,N-dimethyltryptamine | 50 | 45 | 79 | 65 | 107 | 159+ |
| N-methyl-5-hydroxytryptamine | 80 | 71 | 115 | 84 | 120 | 120 |
| 5-methoxytryptamine | 45 | – | 63 | – | 90 | 108+ |
| N,N-dimethyl-5-hydroxytryptamine | 20 | – | 35 | – | 70 | – |
| 5-methoxy-N,N-dimethyltryptamine | 30 | 42 | 55 | 66 | 88 | 86 |
| N-acetyl-5-methoxytryptamine | 90 | – | 96 | – | 100 | – |

*: The values are expressed at % of the activity determined in the absence of added amine.
+: Tested at 2.5 x $10^{-7}$M
Histamine: 1 x $10^{-5}$M; Histamine N-Methyltransferase: after Sephadex G-100 (Table I).

TABLE III.　$K_i$ VALUES FOR INHIBITION OF RAT AND/OR MOUSE BRAIN HISTAMINE N-METHYLTRANSFERASE BY DOPAMINE AND 3 METHYLATED INDOLEAMINES

| Modulator | $K_i$ | Species | Type of Inhibition |
|---|---|---|---|
| None | 5.0 x $10^{-6}$M* | rat, mouse | ---- |
| Dopamine | 4.5 x $10^{-8}$M | rat | non-competitive |
| Dopamine | 4.0 x $10^{-7}$M | mouse | non-competitive |
| N,N-dimethyltryptamine | 7.0 x $10^{-8}$M** | rat | competitive |
| 5-methoxy-N,N-dimethyltryptamine | 1.6 x $10^{-7}$M** | rat | competitive |
| 5-methoxytryptamine | 1.2 x $10^{-6}$M | mouse | competitive |

*$K_m$　(Mean of 13 determinations)

**Determined on the assumption of no HMT stimulation at the low concentrations of the modulator (see Fig. 2).
From (17).

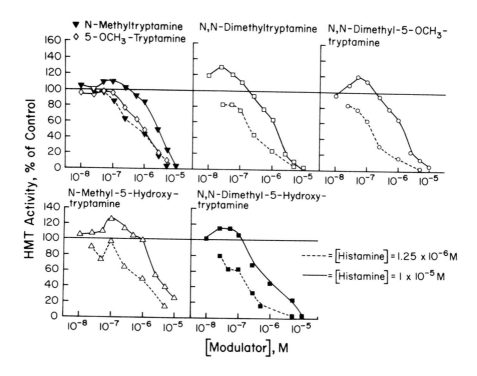

Fig. 2.   Effect of modulators on the activity of rat brain histamine
N-methyltransferase.
The enzyme preparation used was about 150-fold enriched over
the homogenate activity (Sephadex G-100 step, Table I).   It
was incubated at 1 x 10⁻⁵M and 1.25 x 10⁻⁶M histamine (except
for 5-methoxytryptamine, which was incubated only in the presence of 1 x 10⁻⁵M histamine) and in the presence of the indicated concentrations of modulator.   The histamine N-methyltransferase activity ($^{14}$[C]-3-methylhistamine formed in 30
minutes) is expressed as a percentage of the activity observed
in the absence of the modulator (control activity=100%).

inhibition to stimulation (or the reverse) by varying the substrate" (18).   It is
quite likely that, in vivo, similar interactions between neurotransmitters and
methylated trace amines play a significant part in modulating and shaping transmit-
ter-driven neural behaviors.   Studies describing interactions of methylated trace
amines, such as N,N'-dimethyltryptamine, with dopamine and acetylcholine (19,20)
have recently begun to appear and the present findings add to the growing evidence
that the methylated trace amines act as modulators of the actions and of the metabolism of the biogenic amines.

In a further effort to test the notion that the mode of action of methionine sulfoximine is via an elevated methylation of cerebral histamine, we injected $^{3}$[H]-
histamine into the lateral ventricles of methionine sulfoximine-pretreated and con-

trol mice and 15 min later we isolated [3][H]-3-methyl histamine from the brains of the two groups (21). As shown in Fig. 3, the levels of [3][H]-3-methyl histamine were

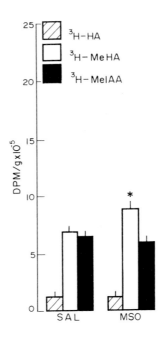

Fig. 3.   Effect of methionine sulfoximine on [3][H]-histamine catabolism in whole mouse brain.
L-methionine-d,l-sulfoximine (170 mg/kg) was injected intraperitoneally 3 hours before sacrifice. [3][H]-histamine (HA) (2 μcuries, 10 μliters) was injected intraventricularly 15 minutes before sacrifice. [3][H]-3-methyl histamine: [3]H-MeHA; [3][H]-3-methylimidazoleacetic acid: [3]H-MeIAA. Results are in d.p.m./g x 10^{-5} (mean ± SEM from 5-6 mice). Total tissue radioactivity (T.R.) is expressed in d.p.m./g x 10^{-6}, also as mean ± SEM. Star denotes a statistically significant difference from saline-injected controls. SAL: saline; MSO: L-methionine-d,l-sulfoximine.

significantly higher in the pretreated animals than in the saline controls. A calculation of the conversion index (22) histamine-- methyl histamine (dpm/g, [3][H]-3-methyl histamine/dpm/nmole, [3][H] histamine) revealed values of 4.5 and 2.2 for the pretreated control groups. Thus, it can now be safely stated that cerebral histamine methylation is increased during the preconvulsant period following the admin-

istration of methionine sulfoximine. Taken together with the results of the in vitro experiments, it is probable that this elevation is mediated by methylated trace
amines. Further research should provide the necessary documentation for this notion.

Indirect support for this notion has come recently from studies of Stramentinoli
and Baldessarini (23) who showed that systemic injections of L-methionine or of SAM
in large acute and repeated doses failed to elevate the endogenous levels of N,N-
dimethyltryptamine and from those of Bidard et al. (24) who showed no change in
striatal 3-0-methyl dopamine levels or in its formation from dopa, following the
administration of SAM $\pm$ dopa. It would seem therefore that only a diminution of
the endogenous SAM pools, as after methionine sulfoximine, coupled to a mediated
activation of the transfer of methyl groups to selected endogenous acceptors (histamine, tRNAs, proteins?) succeeds in perturbing the cellular methylation balance
sufficiently to bring the affected cells into a "preconvulsant" state.

SAH HYDROLASE OF RAT BRAIN
SAH hydrolase has recently been extensively purified from the leaves of the spinach
beet (25), beef liver (26,27) and yellow lupin seeds (28). We have purified the
enzyme from rat brain (29,30) and the procedure, as well as some properties of the
enzyme are reported below. We noted previously that after methionine sulfoximine
SAH hydrolase activity decreases by about 50% in the cerebellum, the brainstem and
the hippocampus (31) and also that the brain activity is several-fold lower than
the corresponding liver and kidney activity in both the rat and the mouse (32).
The purification procedure for SAH hydrolase of rat brain (35 g of starting material) is shown in Table 4. The procedure results in an approximately 2,370-fold
purified protein with a 21% yield. The specific activity of the final preparation
(0.63 µmoles SAH hydrolyzed/min) is somewhat lower than that of the purified beef
liver SAH hydrolase (27). A molecular weight of ca.180,000 daltons,markedly higher
that that of the yellow lupin seed enzyme (MW = 110,000 daltons) (28),was determined by gel exclusion chromatography on Sephadex G-150 and by sucrose density
gradient centrifugation, rabbit muscle aldolase serving as the molecular weight
standard (Fig. 4A and 4B). Upon exposure to 0.1% sodium dodecyl sulfate, the enzyme exhibited one band in 5% polyacrylamide gels, with a molecular weight of a-
bout 45-48,000, by comparison to similarly treated aldolase. Isoelectric focusing
of the purified enzyme revealed a single pI of 5.6. While recently SAH hydrolase
of yellow lupin seeds (28) was shown to form multimers when repeatedly freeze-
thawed, the brain SAH hydrolase tended to form multimers when electrophoresed in
7.5% polyacrylamide gels following exposure to either 0.1% or 1.0% sodium dodecyl
sulfate or, alternatively, when electrophoresed in 5% gels, provided exposure was
to 1% sodium dodecyl sulfate. Aldolase failed to form multimers under any of these

TABLE IV.   PURIFICATION OF RAT BRAIN SAH HYDROLASE

| Fraction | Volume (ml) | Units (nmol/h) | Protein (mg) | Specific activity (nmol/ mg protein) | Yield (%) | Purification |
|---|---|---|---|---|---|---|
| Whole homogenate | 200 | 56,200 | 3,440 | 16 | 100 | 1 |
| 100,00 x g Supernatant | 150 | 40,500 | 765 | 53 | 72 | 3 |
| Sephadex G-200 | 103 | 34,917 | 340 | 103 | 62 | 6 |
| DEAE-Cellulose | 127 | 34,290 | 75 | 457 | 61 | 29 |
| Hydroxylapatite (spheroidal) | 109 | 25,833 | 9.8 | 2,636 | 46 | 165 |
| DEAE-Sephadex A-50 | 130 | 29,900 | 9.1 | 3,285 | 53 | 205 |
| Aminohexyl Sepharose - 4B | 5.3 | 12,068 | 0.32 | 37,950 | 21 | 2,371 |

Enzyme unit: nmol SAH hydrolyzed/h

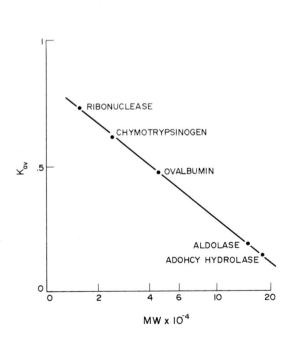

Fig. 4.  The determination of the molecular weight of SAH hydrolase of rat brain.  A) The molecular weight was determined by exclusion chromatography on Sephadex-G-150.  The molecular weights of the standard proteins are plotted in semilog fashion against $K_{av}$;

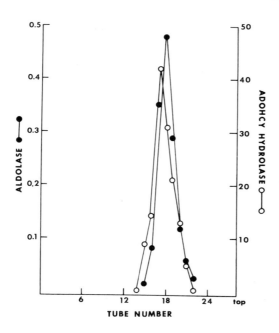

Fig. 4. The determination of
the molecular weight of SAH
hydrolase of rat brain.
B) The molecular weight was
determined by sucrose density gradient centrifugation.
The gradient was 5-25% in
sucrose and contained 1 mM
dithiothreitol.  Centri-
fugation was at 25,000 rpm
in rotor SW. 27 of the Beckman Spinco centrifuge for
14 hours.  Rabbit muscle
aldolase was identified by
its absorbance at 280 nm
and was centrifuged in a
separate tube.  SAH hydrolase activity is expressed
as % of product (inosine)
formed. For details see (32).

conditions and thus differed markedly in this one behavior from the SAH hydrolase
(Fig. 5).  Both aldolase and the hydrolase exhibited an extra band which migrated

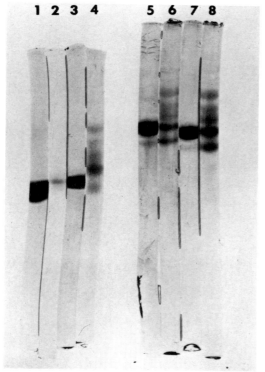

Fig. 5. Polyacrylamide gel e-
lectrophoresis of SAH hydrolase purified from rat brainstem.
SAH hydrolase of highest
purity (after the amino-
hexyl Sepharose-4B step,
Table IV) was electrophoresed in 5% polyacrylamide
gels, pH 7.0, rabbit muscle
aldolase serving as standard. (1,2): aldolase and
SAH hydrolase after exposure
to 0.1% sodium dodecyl sulfate prior to electrophoresis; 3,4:as 1,2 except that
sodium dodecyl sulfate was
19%; 5,6: as 1,2 except that
gels were 7.5% and sodium
dodecyl sulfate was 0.19%;
7,8: as 5,6 except that sodium dodecyl sulfate was 19%.

ahead of the main band in 7.5% gels, suggesting some molecular fragmentation. Non-dialyzed SAH hydrolase was totally inactivated by exposure to $45^{\circ}$C for 7-8 min, while the dialyzed enzyme became inactivated in 5 min. Enzyme activity was totally lost in the presence of 0.05% sodium dodecyl sulfate or 1 x $10^{-4}$M N-ethyl maleimide.

Table 5 shows an apparent $K_m$ value of the enzyme for SAH of 36.6 μmoles/l and two apparent $K_i$ values well below the $K_m$ value, 0.9 μmoles/l for s-5'butyl-deoxyadenosine and 8.4 μmoles/l for d,l-homocysteine. The observed $K_m$ value makes it likely that SAH is close to being saturated with SAH in situ, since the whole brain levels of SAH were recently determined to be 46.3 nmoles/g (31) in the Sprague-Dawley rat used in our experiments. A much lower value of 3.4 nmoles/g (33) was recently determined in the brain of the Wister rat. The $K_m$ value of the brain enzyme is about 3 times higher than that of the enzyme from yellow lupin seeds (28), about equal to that of the enzyme from spinach beet leaves (25) and somewhat lower than the $K_m$ of the enzyme from beef liver (27). SAM and the synthetic cyclohexyl-d,l-homocysteine (34,35) were poor competitive inhibitors of the SAH hydrolase (Table 5). A large number of different compounds was tested as possible inhibitors of brain SAH hydrolase. Tables 6 and 7 list the effective and the ineffective compounds, respectively.

TABLE V.   RAT BRAIN SAH HYDROLASE KINETIC CONSTANTS FOR SAH
AND SOME INHIBITORS

| Compound | $K_m$ of $K_i$ (uM) | Type of inhibition |
|---|---|---|
| SAH | 36.6 | – |
| S-5'-butyl deoxyadenosine | 0.9 | Competitive |
| d,l-homocysteine | 8.4 | " |
| SAM | 25.4 | " |
| Cyclohexyl d,l-homocysteine[+] | 75.0 | " |
| Adenine | 2.5 | Non-competitive |

SAH $V_{max}$: 38.6 μmol/mg/min

Adenine $V_{max_i}$ (1 x $10^{-5}$M): 28.6 μmol/mg/min

+ Prepared according to (34) by Dr. Margaret Clarke

Finally, a subcellular fractionation study of the enzyme (36) (Fig. 6) revealed its enrichment in the high-speed soluble supernatant fraction of brain, while a post-natal development study of the enzyme in several brain regions showed the cerebellar activity to be highest at 8 days (Fig. 7).

In conclusion, we have shown in this brief survey of selected facets of cerebral methylation that this process can be readily affected by the convulsant agent methionine sulfoximine and, in particular, the methylation of cerebral histamine enhanced. The responsible enzyme, histamine N-methyltransferase, was shown to be peculiarly

TABLE VI.   <u>INHIBITION OF RAT BRAIN SAH HYDROLASE</u>[+]

| Compound | Concentration (M) | % Inhibition |
|---|---|---|
| S-5'-butyl deoxyadenosine | $1 \times 10^{-4}$ | 61 |
| Adenine | " | 58 |
| d,1-homocysteine | " | 40 |
| Cyclohexyl-d,1-homocysteine | " | 15 |
| ATP | " | 27 |
| SAM | $5 \times 10^{-4}$ | 51 |
| 1-methyl adenine | " | 44 |
| $N^6$-methyl adenine | " | 24 |
| isopentenyl adenine | " | 15 |
| $N^6,N^6$-dimethyl adenine | " | 12 |
| Polyvinylpyrrolidone | $8 \times 10^{-4}$ | 43 |

[+]SAH concentration: $1.6 \times 10^{-4}$M

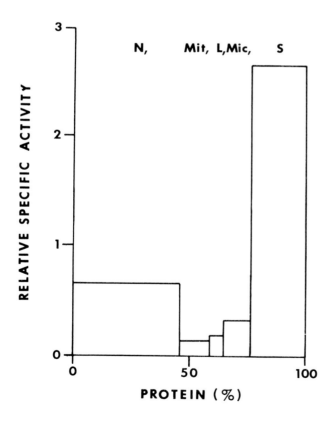

Fig. 6. The subcellular distribution of SAH hydrolase in the adult rat brain. SAH hydrolase activity was determined in the nuclear (N), nerve ending-mitochondrial (Mit), lysosomal (Ly) microsomal (Mic) and soluble (S) fractions obtained by differential centrifugation of rat brain (36) and the percentage of the total activity (N+Mit+Ly+Mic+S) recovered in a given fraction was divided by the percentage of the total protein content of that fraction (abscissa) to give the relative specific activity plotted on the ordinate.

TABLE VII.   COMPOUNDS HAVING NO EFFECT ON BRAIN SAH HYDROLASE

| | |
|---|---|
| cobaltous chloride | benzyl Hcy* |
| calcium chloride | propyl Hcy* |
| mercuric chloride | butyl Hcy* |
| mercurous bromide | t-butyl Hcy* |
| lithium chloride | heptyl-Hcy* |
| lanthanum oxide | pentyl Hcy* |
| cesium chloride | hexyl Hcy* |
| manganous chloride | octyl Hcy* |
| magnesium chloride | l-methionine |
| cuprous sulfate | l-methionine-d, l-sulfoximine |
| lead nitrate | tyramine |
| ferrous sulfate | norepinephrine |
| ferric sulfate | epinephrine |
| zinc acetate | l-cysteine |
| tryptamine | l-cystine |
| N-methyltryptamine | l-ethionine sulfoxide |
| N,N-dimethyltryptamine | 5-methyl cytosine |
| 5-methoxy-N,N-dimethyltryptamine | 7-methyl guanine |
| N-methyl-5-hydroxytryptamine | S-adenosyl-l-ethionine |
| 5-hydroxy tryptamine | histamine |
| 3-methyl histamine | N-methyl histamine |
| N,N'-dimethyl histamine | 1-β -D-arabinofuranosyl adenine** |
| d,l-methionine sulfone | 9-β -D-arabinofuranosyl uracil** |
| α-methyl-dl-methionine | S-5'-isobutyl-5' deoxyadenosine** |
| d,l-methionine sulfoxide | S-adenosyl-5'-deoxy-5'-thioethanol** |
| hypoxanthine | xanthine |
| guanosine | thymine |
| 9-β-D-arabinofuranosyl hypoxanthine** | 2'-0-methyl adenosine |

Test compound concentration = 1 x $10^{-4}$M. Hcy = d,l-homocysteine.

SAH concentration = 1.6 x $10^{-4}$M

*synthesized by Dr. Margaret Clarke according to Ref. 34.

**obtained from Sefochem Ltd., Emek Hayarden, Israel

sensitive in vitro to the action of very small amounts of methylated indoleamines, which were shown to activate the enzyme, but only when it was saturated with its substrate, histamine.  Whether the previously reported in vivo activating effect of methionine sulfoximine on histamine N-methyltransferase is mediated by methylated indoleamines, newly formed in brain cells as part of a general methyl transfer activating response to methionine sulfoximine is not known at this time.

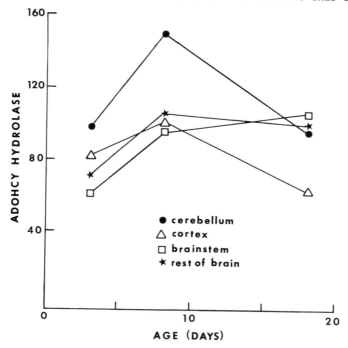

Fig. 7.    The early post-natal development of rat brain SAH hydrolase.
Homogenates of the brain regions indicated were prepared in
0.25 M sucrose and the SAH hydrolase activity determined (32)
at 3,8 and 18 days post-natally.

Since activation of cerebral methylation implies an effective removal of SAH by
brain SAH hydrolase, we examined some of the properties of a 2,370-fold purified
preparation.  The enzyme has a M.W. of about 180,000 daltons; it dissociates into
4 subunits of 45-48,000 daltons, when treated with sodium dodecyl sulfate.  It has
a single pI of 5.6 and it requires SH groups for activity.  Its apparent $K_m$ for SAH
is 36.6 µM, while its apparent $K_i$ for d,1-homocysteine is 8.4 µM.  The most effective inhibitor of brain SAH hydrolase was found to be S-5'-butyl deoxyadenosine
($K_i$ = 0.9 µM).

ACKNOWLEDGEMENT

The research was supported by the U.S. Public Health Service (NINCDS 06294).

REFERENCES

1.  Baldessarini, R.J., _Intern. Rev. Neurobiol._, 18, 41 (1975).

2.  Rosengarten, H. and Friedhoff, A.H., _Schizophrenia Bull._, 2, 90 (1976).

3.  Ordonez, L.A. in "Nutrition and the Brain", Raven Press, New York 205 (1977).

4.  Schatz, R. A. and Sellinger, O.Z., J. Neurochem., 24, 63 (1975).

5.  Lodin, Z. and Kolousek, J., Physiol. Bohemoslov., 7, 87 (1958).

6.  Lamar, C., Jr. and Sellinger, O.Z., Biochem. Pharmacol., 14, 489 (1965).

7.  Sellinger, O.Z., Azcurra, J.M., Ohlsson, W.G., Kohl, H.H. and Zand, R., Fed. Proc., 31, 160 (1972).

8.  Salas, C.E., Ohlsson, W.G. and Sellinger, O.Z., Biochem. Biophys. Res. Commun., 76, 1107 (1977).

9.  Schatz, R.A., Diez Altares, M.C. and Sellinger, O.Z., Trans. Am. Soc. Neurochem., 4, 74 (1973).

10. Schatz, R.A. and Sellinger, O.Z., J. Neurochem., 25, 73 (1975).

11. Maslinski, C., "Agents and Actions", 5, 183 (1975).

12. Thithapandha, A. and Cohn, V.H., Biochem. Pharmacol., 27, 263 (1978).

13. Schwartz, J.-C., Ann. Rev. Pharmacol & Toxicol., 17, 325 (1977).

14. Green, J.P. and Maayani, S., Nature, 269, 163 (1977).

15. Baldessarini, R.J. and Kopin, I.J., J. Neurochem., 13, 769 (1966).

16. Schayer, R.W. and Reilly, M.A., J. Pharmac. Exp. Ther., 187, 34 (1973).

17. Sellinger, O.Z., Schatz, R.A. and Ohlsson, W.G., J. Neurochem., 30, 437, (1978).

18. Reiner, J.M. in "Behavior of Enzyme Systems", Burgess Publ. Co. Minneapolis, Minnesota, 176 (1959).

19. Haubrich, D.R. and Wang, P.F.L., Brain Res., 131, 158 (1977).

20. Waldmeier, P.C. and Maitre, L., Psychopharmacology, 52, 137 (1977).

21. Schatz, R.A., Frye, K. and Sellinger, O.Z., J. Pharmac. Exptl. Therap., 1978, in press.

22. Verdiere, M., Rose, C. and Schwartz., J.-C., Brain Res., 129, 197 (1977).

23. Stramentinoli, G. and Baldessarini, R.J., submitted for publication, (1978).

24. Bidard, J.-N., Darmenton, P., Cronenberger, L. and Pacheco, H., J. Pharmacol. (Paris) 8, 83 (1977).

25. Poulton, J.E. and Butt, V.S., Arch. Biochem. & Biophys., 172, 135 (1976).

26. Palmer, J.L. and Abeles, R.H., J. Biol. Chem., 251, 5817 (1976).

27. Chiang, P.K., Richards, H.H. and Cantoni, G.L., Mol. Pharmac., 13, 939 (1977).

28. Guaranowski, A. and Pawelkiewicz, J., Eur. J. Biochem., 80, 517 (1977).

29. Schatz, R.A., Vunnam, C.R. and Sellinger, O.Z., Trans. Am. Soc. Neurochem., 8, 181 (1977).

30. Schatz, R.A., Vunnam, C.R. and Sellinger, O.Z., <u>Trans. Am. Soc. Neurochem.</u>, 9, 160 (1978).

31. Schatz, R.A., Vunnam, C.R. and Sellinger, O.Z., <u>Neurochem. Res.</u>, 2, 27 (1977).

32. Schatz, R.A., Vunnam, C.R. and Sellinger, O.Z., <u>Life Sci.</u>, 20, 375 (1977).

33. Eloranta, T.O., <u>Biochem. J.</u>, 166, 521 (1977).

34. Armstrong, M.D. and Lewis, J.D., <u>J. Org. Chem.</u>, 16, 749 (1951).

35. Kolenbrander, H.M., <u>Can. J. Chem.</u>, 47, 3271 (1969).

36. Sellinger, O.Z. and deBalbian Verster, F., <u>J.Biol. Chem.</u>, 237, 2836 (1972).

# Studies on Indoleamine N-Methyltransferase, an Enzyme Possibly Involved in Psychotic Disorders

**Raffaele Porta, Carla Esposito and Gennaro Della Pietra**

Department of Biochemistry, 1st Medical School, University of Naples, via Costantinopoli 16, 80138 Naples, Italy

In the wide field of methyltransferases, there has been a particular interest since 1960 on the isolation and characterization of enzymes involved in biogenic amine metabolism. Owing to technological improvements in protein purification, the initial researches emphasizing non-specifically methylating enzymes were followed by identification of several completely differentiated 0- and N-methylating activities (1). However, most of these enzymes exist in multiple molecular forms within both different species and various organs of a given animal. Table 1 gives a resume of the enzymes methylating biogenic amines in mammal tissues.

TABLE I.   ENZYMES METHYLATING BIOGENIC AMINES IN MAMMAL TISSUES

---

Phenylethanolamine N-methyltransferase (PNMT)

methylates amino nitrogen of catecholamines

Catechol 0-methyltransferase (COMT)

methylates phenolic oxygen of catecholamines

Hydroxyindole 0-methyltransferase (HIOMT)

methylates phenolic oxygen of indoleamines

Indoleamine N-methyltransferase (INMT)

methylates amino nitrogen of indoleamines

Histamine N-methyltransferase (HMT)

methylates imidazole nitrogen of histamine

---

*Abbreviations used: SAM, S-adenosylmethionine; MTHF, methyltetrahydrofolate; INMT, indoleamine N-methyltransferase; PNMT, phenylethanolamine N-methyltransferase; COMT, catechol 0-methyltransferase; HIOMT, hydroxyindole 0-methyltransferase; HMT, histamine N-methyltransferase; DMT, N,N-dimethyltryptamine; SAH, S-adenosylhomocysteine; CPZ, chlorpromazine; nor$_1$ CPZ, mono-N-demethylchlorpromazine; nor$_2$ CPZ, di-N-demethylchlorpromazine; LSD, lysergic acid diethylamide; DBN, 2,3,4,6,7,8-hexahydropyrrolo [1,2 -a]pyrimidine; PCMB, p-chloromercuribenzoic acid; MTA, methylthioadenosine; TLC, thin-layer chromatography; GLC, gas-liquid chromatography.

The enzyme activities listed, as all the known methyltransferases (i.e., tRNA methylases, protein methylases) require S-adenosylmethionine (SAM) as the methyl donor. The only exception is the enzyme catalyzing methionine synthesis from homocysteine which is methyltetrahydrofolate (MTHF)-dependent (2).

In 1972, experimental evidence was published on MTHF-dependent N-methylation of dopamine, tryptamine and phenylethylamine; Laduron et al. (3) obtained dopamine N-methylation in vitro by using an enzyme from rat brain requiring MTHF as the methyl donor. Furthermore, Hsu and Mandell (4) described tryptamine and phenylethylamine N-methylation employing the same enzyme source and MTHF as methyl donor, while Banerjee and Snyder found in various mammalian and avian tissues MTHF-dependent indoleamine and phenylethylamine N-methylases (5). These findings prompted several authors to consider MTHF as the most specific physiological methyl donor for N-methylation in brain of various biogenic amines.

Recently a difference has been noted in the reaction product when the methyl donor used in the enzymatic in vitro assay was MTHF instead of SAM. In 1975, it was reported (6,7,8) the enzymatic conversion of MTHF to methylenetetrahydrofolate by means of reductase with a subsequent non-enzymatic condensation of deriving formaldehyde with dopamine or tryptamine. The final reaction products were identified as 6,7-dihydroxy-1,2,3,4-tetrahydroisoquinoline and 1,2,3,4-tetrahydro-β-carboline. These data show that MTHF does not participate in the transmethylation process but it is a simple substrate of a specific reductase.

Concerning SAM-dependent enzymes, indoleamine N-methyltransferase (INMT), first considered as a non-specific N-methylase (9), has been recently a subject of particular interest because of its possible involvement in schizophrenic syndromes. This enzyme, demonstrated in various human tissues (lung, blood, cerebrospinal fluid) (10,11,12), seems to be present at fairly high activity in rabbit lung (9). Widely extended studies demonstrated that INMT methylates tryptamine to N-methyltryptamine; this goes on to N,N-dimethyltryptamine (DMT). Serotonin, N-methylserotonin, O-methylserotonin and O-methyl-N-methylserotonin are also good substrates for INMT.

Various hypotheses were proposed for the biological significance of INMT. Although the general opinion is that INMT has a regulatory function with regard to tryptamine and serotonin inactivation, a specific action on N-methylated indoleamines cannot be excluded (13).

In conclusion, the psychotomimetic properties of dimethylated indoleamines and their possible biosynthesis give rise to interest in present biochemical researches on molecular and catalytic characteristics of INMT.

BIOCHEMICAL STUDIES ON INMT

## Purification procedure

Based on reported studies (14,15), the following purification steps for rabbit lung INMT seem the most effective: 1) tissue homogenization with 5 vol. (w/v) of 10 mM potassium phosphate buffer, pH 7.3 followed by discarding pellet after centrifugation of the mixture; (2) supernatant saturation with ammonium sulfate: the proteins precipitating between 50-75% saturation contain INMT activity; (3) anion-exchange chromatography (DEAE-cellulose or DE-Sephadex) at pH 7.0 with elution by ionic strength gradient; (4) gel filtration; (5) preparative electrofocusing.

## Enzyme assay and product analysis

The activity of INMT is assayed by incubating the enzyme at 37°C and pH 7.9 in the presence of the two substrates (indoleamine and SAM). The reaction is stopped by addition of borate buffer, pH 11.0 and the methylated products are extracted by ethyl acetate from the reaction mixture (15). Then, the amount of methylated indoleamines can be determined by the following methods:

1) radiometric method (15): when the enzymatic assay is performed by using as substrate SAM labeled in the methyl group, the reaction products are quantified by counting the radioactivity in an aliquot of the organic phase after extraction of the reaction mixture.

2) TLC-fluorometric method (16,17): after thin-layer chromatography (TLC) of an aliquot of the ethyl acetate extract, the spot(s) isographic with the standard (methylated derivatives of serotonin) are detected fluorometrically by derivatization with o-phthalaldehyde.

3) GLC method: the organic phase is submitted to GLC after derivatization of the amino and indole nitrogens of indoleamines (18) or of the hydroxyl group of serotonin derivatives (16). A GLC procedure for separation and quantitation of tryptamine and N-methyltryptamine without derivatization has been recently developed (19).

## Distribution and heterogeneity

An involvement in this particularly active serotonin metabolism of the rabbit lung is the probable meaning of the large amount of INMT in this organ. Nevertheless, INMT activity has also been demonstrated in other tissues of various organisms including human. With regard to the nervous system, different results reported by various laboratories (10,17,20,21) lead us to conclude that the INMT present in the brain is not very significant. Similarly, the data indicating the existence of heterogeneous forms of INMT in different tissues (22) are not definitive; this question needs further study. In this regard, careful consideration must be given to the recent findings (23) showing the existence in the rabbit lung of two molecular forms of INMT which differ in charge properties.

## Molecular and catalytic properties

As illustrated in Table 2, the rabbit lung enzyme exhibits higher affinity for N-methyltryptamine than for other indoleamine substrates.  Table 3 demonstrates that

TABLE II.  AFFINITY OF RABBIT LUNG INMT TOWARD VARIOUS SUBSTRATES

| Substrate | $K_m$, M |
|---|---|
| S-Adenosylmethionine | $5 \times 10^{-5}$ |
| Tryptamine | $4 \times 10^{-4}$ |
| N-Methyltryptamine | $1 \times 10^{-4}$ |
| Serotonin | $1 \times 10^{-3}$ |
| N-Methylserotonin | $4 \times 10^{-4}$ |
| O-Methylserotonin | $4 \times 10^{-4}$ |
| O-Methyl-N-methylserotonin | $4 \times 10^{-4}$ |

INMT from human lung has $K_m$ values for indoleamines higher than those observed with the rabbit enzyme (10).  Moreover, the results of experiments carried out with the synthetic substrate 1-methyltryptamine ($K_m$, $4.25 \times 10^{-4}$ M) (24) indicate that the methyl group present on the indole nitrogen does not influence INMT catalysis.

TABLE III.  AFFINITY OF HUMAN LUNG INMT TOWARD SOME INDOLEAMINES

| Substrate | $K_m$, M |
|---|---|
| Tryptamine | $1.2 \times 10^{-3}$ |
| N-Methyltryptamine | $2.8 \times 10^{-4}$ |
| Serotonin | $2.3 \times 10^{-3}$ |
| N-Methylserotonin | $5.7 \times 10^{-4}$ |

Several authors report an optimal pH of 7.9, determined in phosphate buffer for in-doleamine N-methylation.  Thus, substrate binding appears to occur at pH values a-bove the enzyme isoelectric point ($\sim$5.0).  Finally, recent gel filtration experi-ments using various calibration proteins reveal a low molecular weight for rabbit lung INMT (15).

## Reaction mechanism

From the various studies performed, it can be concluded that INMT reaction occurs in three stages; the first of which is the reversible formation of an INMT-SAM complex. Only this complex would be capable of binding the indoleamine and methylating it, with subsequent release of products. Furthermore, from experiments carried out with 1-methyltryptamine, it can be deduced that indoleamine interacts with exposed hydrophobic binding sites furnished by the enzymatic protein. The following data support for INMT an "Ordered Bi Bi" mechanism: 1) the $K_m$ value for SAM is clearly lower than the value measured for various indoleamines; 2) INMT preincubation in the presence of SAM increases the reaction rate (25); 3) the inhibition by S-adenosylhomocysteine (SAH) is more consistent when the enzyme is preincubated with SAM and SAH; this disappears after reaction mixture dialysis (25); 4) protein binding with competitive inhibitors of indoleamines does not occlude the SAM active site (15).

## Inhibition studies

INMT studies aimed at discovering possible enzyme inhibitors were performed both to determine chemical and physical properties of the enzyme active site and to explain the reaction mechanism. If more significant experimental data were obtained for an anomalous INMT function in some mental disease, great interest would be aroused for the possibility of a therapeutic treatment by means of enzyme inhibitors.

Since the subject seems of possible value, the main INMT inhibitors now known are listed; first, possible physiological inhibitors and then synthetic inhibitors having demonstrated pharmacological interest.

a) Physiological inhibitors

1) S-adenosylhomocysteine (SAH)
This substance, derived from SAM by demethylation _in vivo_, is capable of exerting an effective "product" inhibition on INMT, as on all SAM-dependent methyltransferases.
SAH shows a competitive type of inhibition with respect to SAM and a non-competitive type of inhibition toward indoleamines, with a $K_i$ value of about $1.0 \times 10^{-5}$ M (25). According to enzyme preincubation experiments _in vitro_ in the presence of SAH, a reaction mechanism of "Ordered Bi Bi" type has been suggested for INMT (25). Moreover, dialysis experiments also showed SAH inhibition reversibility.

Since SAH inhibitory effectiveness is extended to all methyltransferases, some investigations were carried out on various analogs of SAH in order to obtain a more specific INMT inhibitor (26). The SAH analogs synthesized involved modifications on the base, on the sugar or on the amino acidic chain. The results obtained demonstrated that the structural characteristics necessary for SAH inhibitory action were the following: a) the homocysteine in L-configuration; b) the amino and carboxyl groups of L-homocysteine; c) the sulfur atom; d) the three carbon distance between the sulfur atom and the terminal amino and carboxyl groups; e) the adenine amino group; f) the hydroxyl group in ribose 2' position. Neither the nitrogen atom of the aromatic ring nor the hydroxyl group in the sugar 3' position were essential for inhibitory effectiveness.

These findings helped to obtain new SAH analogs with more specific inhibitory properties towards various methyltransferases acting on biogenic amines (Table 4).  It

TABLE IV.  $K_i$ VALUES (µM) of SAH AND SOME OF ITS ANALOGS USING VARIOUS METHYL-
TRANSFERASES AS ENZYME SOURCE

| Inhibitor | INMT | COMT | PNMT | HMT | HIOMT |
|---|---|---|---|---|---|
| SAH | 8.65 | 36.3 | 29.0 | 18.1 | 18.5 |
| 3-Deaza-SAH | 26.60 | 80.6 | 81.1 | 59.2 | 229.0 |
| $N^6$-Methyl-3-deaza-SAH | 70.20 | – | 1243.0 | – | – |
| 3'-Deoxy-SAH | 51.90 | 138.0 | 42.7 | 2070.0 | – |

is interesting to point out that $N^6$-methyl-3-deaza-SAH exerts a significant inhibition exclusively on INMT; this requires further pharmacological studies.

2) N,N-Dimethyltryptamine and bufotenin

Dimethylated products of tryptamine and serotonin exert an inhibitory activity on INMT less than the one produced by SAH at similar concentration; it is of the non-competitive type with respect both to SAM and indoleamine (10,27).  This kinetic data would indicate an allosteric mechanism in the regulation of INMT activity.  The $K_i$ value of DMT seems to be about $10^{-4}$ M.  However, although this inhibition could have in vivo significance for preventing production of hallucinogenic substances, it is noteworthy that it does not have any pharmacological interest.

3) Dialyzable peptide factor

Even through the first research on indoleamine N-methylation, dialysis resulted to produce a different INMT activation in relation to the enzyme biological source. Narasimhachari and Lin in 1974 (28) found a considerable INMT-inhibiting activity in bovine pineal extracts.  The dialyzability, the positive reaction with ninhydrin and the retention on a cationic-exchange resin indicated that the partially purified factor had peptide characteristics with possible neurohormone functions.

Moreover, Marzullo et al. in 1977 (29) purified via Sephadex G-25 from a new-born rabbit brain two peptides (I, mol.wt.1500; II, mol. wt.1300) acting as lung INMT inhibitors; these were inactivated by trypsin digestion. Treatment with carboxy-peptidase (carboxypeptidase A, type II) produced from peptide II a less active frag-ment strongly retained by Sephadex G-25. Thus, form I was considered as the native peptide, subsequently altered during the purification procedure. The peptide inhib-itory activity was also shown in other rabbit tissues (Table 5).

Further significant experiments performed by the same authors suggested the exist-ence of an INMT control in vivo. In fact, i.v. injected tryptamine did not produce

in rabbits detectable amounts of N-methyltryptamine or DMT, even when high doses of MAO inhibitors were given (but here tryptamine accumulation mainly was observed in the lung). Moreover, INMT activity from treated rabbits could be shown only after dialysis of tissue extracts.

In view of the results described, it can be assumed that an abnormal production of psychotomimetic catabolites in some schizophrenic syndromes is related to an al-tered turnover of such peptide factor.

4) Methylthioadenosine

Methylthioadenosine (MTA), a secondary product of the polyamine biosynthetic path-way, derives from the transpropylamination reaction of decarboxylated SAM and pu-trescine or spermidine. This compound, having an inhibitory activity on various methyltransferases, suggests a metabolic relation between polyamine synthesis and transmethylation processes.

A MTA inhibiting action in vitro recently has been found with respect to INMT (23). This inhibition, competitive for SAM and non-competitive toward indoleamine, seems to be similar to the one exerted by SAH ($K_i$ is about $0.7 \times 10^{-3}$ M).

b) Synthetic inhibitors

1) Phenothiazines and derivatives

In 1962 Axelrod (9) first demonstrated an inhibitory effect of chlorpromazine (CPZ) on rabbit lung INMT. The low $I_{50}$ value for CPZ suggested the possibility of an in vivo enzyme interaction with the antipsychotic drug.

In 1974 (30), the action of phenothiazines on INMT was investigated more carefully and the research was extended to the metabolites of CPZ. Among the 168 theoretical-ly possible CPZ metabolites, mono-N-demethylchlorpromazine (nor$_1$CPZ), di-N-demethyl-chlorpromazine (nor$_2$CPZ) and the corresponding hydroxylated compounds and sulfoxides were isolated from microsomes of rat, rabbit and human liver cells. These studies showed nor$_1$CPZ and nor$_2$CPZ N-methylation in vitro by rabbit lung INMT to CPZ and nor$_1$CPZ respectively. Another CPZ metabolite, 7-hydroxy-nor$_1$CPZ, acts as an ef-fective substrate for INMT, while 7-hydroxy-8-methoxy-nor$_1$CPZ, 7-hydroxy-8-methoxy-nor$_2$CPZ, nor$_1$CPZ and nor$_2$CPZ sulfoxides and 7-hydroxysulfoxides are less active.

In view of these findings, it was hypothesized that the antipsychotic properties of CPZ are the result of action by its metabolites.

In 1976 (31) some substances (norperazine, norprochlorperazine, amoxapine, $nor_1$ promazine, nortriptyline), structurally related to CPZ demethylated products, were examined in order to determine a possible structure-function relationship. Of these compounds, norperazine ($K_m$, $3 \times 10^{-4}$ M), norprochlorperazine ($K_m$, $2 \times 10^{-4}$ M) and amoxapine ($K_m$, $3 \times 10^{-4}$ M) particularly, appeared to be effective substrates for INMT.

Finally, a recent investigation (32) has indicated that some CPZ analogs show inhibitory activity for INMT without acting as substrates. Among these substances (7,8-dihydroxy-CPZ; 7,8-dioxy-CPZ; 7-hydroxy-CPZ; 8-hydroxy-CPZ; 7,8-diacetoxy-CPZ), 7,8-dihydroxy-CPZ and 7,8-dioxy-CPZ have a high inhibitory effect ($K_i$, $10^{-4}$ M) by a non-competitive mechanism.

The antipsychotic effectiveness of several compounds among those mentioned here has not been investigated, although there should be interest in this.

2) DBN (2,3,4,6,7,8-hexahydropyrrolo[1,2-a]pyrimidine)

DBN appears at present to be the most potent and specific inhibitor of INMT (33). Its activity has been demonstrated by experiments with INMT from human lung and liver, rabbit lung and rat liver, using almost all possible indoleamine substrates. The kinetic parameters, determined by using rabbit lung enzyme, showed that DBN is a noncompetitive inhibitor with respect to the indoleamine with a $K_i$ value of $2 \times 10^{-6}$ M. The inhibitory specificity was shown by the experiments carried out with PNMT and HMT. In fact, these methyltransferase activities proved quite indifferent to DBN influence.

DBN activity was investigated in vivo by injecting i.v. (ear vein) in male rabbits 0.3-30 mg/kg of drug. Lung enzyme activity was reduced to 25% of control values after 10 min and it was hardly demonstrable after 4 hr. Furthermore, when DBN was given orally as the free-base or the fumarate salt, an INMT activity decrease of 70% was observed after four days and its disappearance after eight days. Another dose of the drug was supplied orally at the time of i.v. injection of $[^{14}C]$-N-methyltryptamine and pheniprazine (in order to prevent indoleamine oxidation). The findings obtained showed a decreased production of lung DMT in DBN-treated rabbits with respect to the controls, while a simultaneous lowering of blood DMT was observed (1-3 ng/ml in comparison with 22-34 ng/ml for the controls).

In conclusion DBN, because of its inhibitory effectiveness, specificity and apparent absence of collateral effects, requires further studies in order to control all the suitable characteristics for a possible therapeutic use.

3)   Aliphatic diamines

The discovery in 1977 (15) of an inhibitory activity exerted by some aliphatic
diamines is significant in the explanation of the reaction mechanism of indoleamine N-methylation.  The kinetic pattern of INMT inhibition (uncompetitive toward
SAM and competitive toward tryptamine) by the two most active diamine inhibitors,
1,8-diaminooctane ($K_i$, 8 x $10^{-4}$ M) and 1,7-diaminoheptane ($K_i$, 1.8 x $10^{-3}$ M), suggested an "Ordered Bi Bi" reaction mechanism with SAM as the first substrate bound.
Moreover, in view of these findings, it cannot be stated that the enzyme site for
diamine is identical to the one involved in indoleamine binding, although it is
possible there is a diamine structural arrangement rather similar to the one of
the indoleamine molecule both in the distance between polar groups and in the width
of the hydrophobic area.

4)   p-Chloromercuribenzoic acid (PCMB)

PCMB allowed proof of the presence of essential thiol groups in the INMT molecule.
In 1962 Axelrod (9) first showed the inhibitory action of PCMB on the enzymatic N-
methylation of serotonin; he reported an $I_{50}$ value of about $10^{-5}$ M.  Further recent experiments (23) with purified INMT preparations indicate an $I_{50}$ value of 2 x
$10^{-6}$ M in the case of tryptamine N-methylation.  However, the inhibitory effect disappears when the enzyme is incubated in the presence of such reducing agents as
dithiothreitol.

5)   Further inhibitors

In 1976, an extensive investigation was performed (34) to discover new inhibitors
or substrates of INMT purified from rabbit lung.  The results showed the inhibitory properties of 2-(2-aminoethyl)-5,6-dichlorobenzimidazole ($I_{50}$, 2.6 x $10^{-5}$ M),
5,6-dichloro-2-benzimidazole ($I_{50}$, 3.2 x $10^{-4}$ M), 2-(3-aminopropyl)-5,6-dichloro-
benzimidazole ($I_{50}$, 3.2 x $10^{-4}$ M), 2-aminomethyl-5,6-dichlorobenzimidazole ($I_{50}$,
5.1 x $10^{-4}$ M), N-(2-aminoethyl)-pyrrolidine ($I_{50}$, 2.8 x $10^{-4}$ M).  Kinetic studies
carried out with the first of the mentioned compounds showed a non-competitive type
of inhibition toward both substrates with a $K_i$ value of 6 x $10^{-5}$ M.  Moreover, the
same experimental study showed that various substances could act as substrates in
addition to the indoleamines.  The most active compounds are the following (the
effectiveness is expressed as % of methylation with respect to the amount of N-
methyltryptamine methylated under the same conditions):  1,2,3,4-tetrahydro-3-
methylthianaphtheno-[3,2-c]-pyridine (54.3%); 2-2(2,5-dichlorophenyl)-cyclopropyl-
amine (49.2%); 2-phenylmethylpyrrolidine (42.5%).

INMT INVOLVEMENT IN SCHIZOPHRENIC SYNDROMES

Among the various theories for the etiology of schizophrenia, particular attention has been addressed in recent years to possible alteration in the CNS serotonin and tryptophan metabolism.

Experiments performed with various hallucinogenic compounds [e.g., lysergic acid diethylamide (LSD), bufotenin or N,N-dimethyltryptamine] have allowed comparison of the symptoms produced by such substances with those present in various mental diseases. In this context, the possibility of anomalous functions of INMT with a consequent alteration of indoleamine catabolism is of interest. In fact, exogenous DMT, if parenterally introduced in normal subjects, causes a model psychosis (10), giving rise to the hypothesis that the typical symptoms of schizophrenia can be due to an abnormal production of DMT.

Although several experimental data have been collected, the mechanism of the psycho-tomimetic action of DMT is still unknown. The conclusions of these studies are the following: 1) DMT is a potent but short-acting inhibitor of serotonin oxidative deamination (35); 2) DMT increases the accumulation of dopamine and 3-methoxytyra-mine synthesized from dihydroxyphenylalanine (35); 3) DMT causes a considerable de-crease of 3,4-dihydroxyphenylacetic acid with respect to homovanillic acid (35); 4) DMT, as LSD, specifically antagonizes serotonin excitation of single neurons and only rarely antagonizes glutamate effects (36). Finally, it has been recently re-ported that DMT acts on the cat visual system, causing a decrease in amplitude of the response evoked by optic chiasm stimulation (37).

As concerns the synthesis in vivo of such psychotomimetic indoleamines, traces of mono-and dimethylated derivatives are generally found in human urine and sometimes in blood (38): the excretion seems independent of diet or of bacterial action. Fur-ther studies, not yet confirmed nor sufficiently supported by experimental evidence, indicate that in patients with various mental diseases the 24-hr urinary DMT is higher than in other patients or in controls. Although the cerebral origin of DMT is uncertain, there is no doubt about the presence in human lung and in plate-lets of a SAM-dependent INMT capable of forming DMT and bufotenin from tryptamine and serotonin respectively. The most significant results obtained in the last years are chronologically as follows:

1) Narasimhachari et al. (39) in 1972 measured INMT activity (using serotonin or 0-methylserotonin as substrate) from blood of eleven controls, seven acute schizo-phrenics and eighteen chronic schizophrenics during acute episodes. The studies demonstrated that: a) in control blood samples there was no evidence of bufotenin or 0-methyl-DMT produced by INMT activity; b) six of the seven samples obtained from acute schizophrenics demonstrated bufotenin and 0-methyl-N,N-dimethylserotonin production.

2) In 1972, further studies of Narasimhachari et al. (40) demonstrated that four

of six chronic schizophrenics, drug-free for twenty eight days and on an unrestrict-
ed diet, seldom eliminated bufotenin and DMT in their urine; the appearance of these
compounds was in agreement with behavior worsening.  In contrast, the seven controls
did not excrete them, even when submitted to a serotonin-rich diet (DMT and bufotenin levels were never higher than 1-3 μg in a 24-hr urine sample.)

3)  Experiments performed by Wyatt et al. (38) in 1973 on controls, acute schizophrenics, chronic schizophrenics and psychotically depressed patients, did not show
any difference in plasma DMT content, while a higher INMT activity was noted in
platelets from schizophrenics than from controls (41).  Since they found that dialysis of enzymatic extracts from controls restored the values obtained with the
platelets extracts of schizophrenics, these authors suggest that the difference due
to a low molecular weight INMT inhibitor, present in the controls platelets but
absent or diminished in schizophrenic ones.

4)  Narasimhachari and Lin (30) in 1974 showed that chlorpromazine N-demethylated
metabolites are good substrates for INMT.  This is in accordance both with the antipsychotic properties of chlorpromazine and with a possible INMT involvement in
schizophrenic syndrome pathogenesis.

5)  Axelsson and Nordgren (42) in 1974 did not find any methylated indoleamines
present in plasma from schizophrenics or controls, deducing thereby that the different results previously obtained by other authors, who used whole blood samples,
implied the presence of these substances in the blood cells.

6)  It is noteworthy, among the most recent data, the result obtained by Oon and
Rodnight (43) in 1977, who showed a higher DMT content in 24-hr urines from patients
with various mental diseases than from controls.

With regard to possible role of MTHF in schizophrenic syndrome etiology, although
MTHF does not participate in indoleamine transmethylation processes, it has been
shown to contribute to the formation of 1,2,3,4-tetrahydro-β-carboline compounds
which are very similar to the notoriously psychotomimetic alkaloids harmine and
harmaline.  In this respect one case of "folate-responsive schizophrenia" in an
adolescent girl has been recently described: the patient showed typical schizophrenic symptoms together with a deficiency of genetically determined methylenetetrahydrofolate reductase activity.  The enzyme defect involves a typical homo-
cysteinuria caused by inefficient homocysteine re-methylation to methionine (44).

A further interesting involvement recently hypothesized for INMT refers to the results followed to the measure of plasma enzyme activity during the various sleep
phases.  The obtained findings evinced significant fluctuations of enzymatic activity in accordance with a possible INMT influence on the maintenance of mental
activity in the NREM sleep stage (45).

REFERENCES

1. Axelrod, J. and Vessel, E.S., Mol. Pharmacol., 6, 78 (1970).

2. Cantoni, G.L., Ann. Rev. Biochem., 44, 435 (1975).

3. Laduron, P., Nature New Biol., 238, 212 (1972).

4. Hsu, L.L. and Mandell, A.J., Life Sci., 13, 874 (1973).

5. Banerjee, S.P. and Snyder, S.H., Science, 182, 74 (1973).

6. Meller, E., Rosengarten, H., Friedhoff, A.J., Stebbins, R.B. and Silber, R., Science, 187, 171 (1975).

7. Taylor, R.T. and Hanna, M.L., Life Sci., 17, 111 (1975).

8. Pearson, A.G.M. and Turner, A.J., Nature, 258, 173 (1975).

9. Axelrod, J., J. Pharmacol. Exp. Therap., 138, 28 (1962).

10. Mandel, L.R., Ahn, H.S., Vandenheuvel, W.J.A. and Walker, R.W., Biochem. Pharmacol., 21, 1197 (1972).

11. Wyatt, R.J., Saavedra, J.M. and Axelrod, J., Am. J. Psychiatry, 130, 754 (1973).

12. Narasimhachari, N. and Lin, R.L., Brain Res., 87, 126 (1975).

13. Sellinger, O.Z., Schatz, R.A. and Ohlsson, N.G., J. Neurochem., 30, 437 (1978).

14. Mandel, L.R., Biochem. Pharmacol., 20, 712 (1971).

15. Porta, R., Camardella, M., Esposito, C., and Della Pietra, G., Biochem. Biophys. Res. Commun., 77, 1196 (1977).

16. Narasimhachari, N., Lin, R.L., Plaut, J. and Leiner, K., J. Chromatogr., 86, 123 (1973).

17. Narasimhachari, N. and Lin, R.L., Biochem. Med., 11, 171 (1974).

18. Christian, S.T., Benington, F., Morin, R.D. and Corbett, L., Biochem. Med., 14, 191 (1975).

19. Porta, R., Esposito, C., Camardella, M. and Della Pietra, G., J. Chromatogr., 154, 279 (1978).

20. Bhikharidas, B., Mann, L.R.B. and McLeod, W.R., J. Neurochem., 24, 203 (1975).

21. Gomes, U.R., Neethling, A.C. and Shanley, B.C., J. Neurochem., 27, 701 (1976).

22. Thithapanda, A., Biochem. Biophys. Res. Commun., 47, 301 (1972).

23. Porta, R., Esposito, C., Camardella, M., and Della Pietra, G., unpublished data.

24. Lin, R.L. and Narasimhachari, N., Biochem. Pharmacol., 24, 1239 (1975).

25. Lin, R.L., Narasimhachari, N. and Himwich, H.E., Biochem. Biophys. Res. Commun., 54, 751 (1973).

26. Borchardt, R.T., Biochem. Pharmacol., 24, 1542 (1975).

27. Krause, R.R. and Domino, E.F., Res. Commun. Chem. Pathol. Pharmacol., 9, 359 (1974).

28. Narasimhachari, N., Lin, R.L. and Himwich, H.E., Res. Commun. Chem. Pathol. Pharmacol., 9, 375 (1974).

29. Marzullo, G., Rosengarten, H. and Friedhoff, A.J., Life Sci., 20, 775 (1977).

30. Narasimhachari, N., and Lin, R.L., Res. Commun. Chem. Pathol. Pharmacol., 8, 341 (1974).

31. Narasimhachari, N. and Lin, R.L., Psychopharmacology Commun., 2, 27 (1976).

32. Sangiah, S., and Domino, E.F., Res. Commun. Chem. Pathol. Pharmacol., 16, 389 (1977).

33. Mandel, L.R., Biochem. Pharmacol., 24, 2251 (1976).

34. Domino, E.F., Arch. Intern. Pharmac. et Ther., 221, 75 (1976).

35. Waldmeier, P.C. and Maitre, L., Psychopharmacology, 52, 137 (1977).

36. Bradley, P.B. and Briggs, I., Br. J. Pharmacol., 50, 345 (1974).

37. Moore, R.H., Hatada, K. and Domino, E.F., Neuropharmacology, 15, 535 (1976).

38. Wyatt, R.J., Mandel, L.R., Ahn, H.S., Walker, R.W. and Vandenheuvel, W.J.A., Psychopharmacologia, 31, 265 (1973).

39. Narasimhachari, N., Plaut, J. and Himwich, H.E., Life Sci., 11, 221 (1972).

40. Narasimhachari, N., Avalos, J., Fujimori, M. and Himwich, H.E., Biol. Psychiat., 5, 311 (1972).

41. Wyatt, R.J., Saavedra, J.M., Belmaker, R., Cohen, S. and Pollin, W., Am. J. Psychiat., 130, 1359 (1973).

42. Axelssen, S. and Nordgren, L., Life Sci., 14, 1261 (1974).

43. Oon, M.C.H. and Rodnight, R., Biochem. Med., 18, 410 (1977).

44. Rodnight, R., Nature, 258, 108 (1975).

45. Strahilevitz, M., Othmer, E., Narasimhachari, N., Othmer, S.C. and Jacobs, L.S., Biol. Psychiatry, 12, 171 (1977).

# Action of S-Adenosylmethionine on the Hypothalamic-Hypophyseal-Prolactin Axis

## V. Rizza, N. Ragusa, G. Clementi, A. Prato and U. Scapagnini

Department of Pharmacology, School of Medicine, University of Catania, Catania, Italy

Due to its multiple action on several components of the neuro-endocrine axis (NEA), SAM can play an active role in the basal or the phasic regulation of endocrine param— eters. In this paper, we first review a theoretical model which can account for the regulatory action of SAM. Next we summarize some of our studies of the activity of SAM on the single components of a specific NEA. The basic scheme representing the theoretical levels of activity of SAM upon the single components of NEA is il-lustrated in Fig. 1. At the level of the hypothalamus, a modification of various

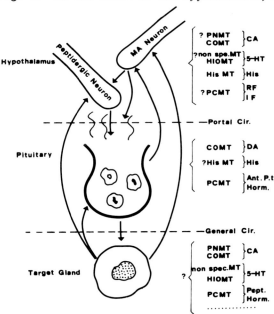

Fig. 1. Schematic representation of the possible mechanisms of action of SAM-dependent enzymes on neuroendocrine axes.

neurotransmitters, catecholamines (CA), serotin (5-HT) and histamine (H), mainly implicated at a central level in the modulation of the hypothalamic releasing or inhibiting hormones (HRF-HIF) (I) could be produced by a SAM-dependent change in

the activity of the key enzymes, catechol 0-methyltransferase (COMT), 5-hydroxyin-
dole 0-methyltransferase (HIMT) and histamine methyltransferase (HMT). Furthermore,
the synthesis and metabolic transformation of the HRF-HIF can also be modified by
changes in the activity of the SAM-dependent enzyme, protein carboxy transferase
(CPT). A direct action at the pituitary level can also be postulated. In other
words, SAM-dependent changes in COMT and HMT could be responsible for modifications
of the monoaminergic input at the level of the anterior pituitary (AP) cells. A
change in CMT can also produce structural modification of the AP trophines (2,3,4,5).
Finally by its action on the target glands, SAM could bring about a peripheral modification in the state of activity of NEA.

In the present paper we will focus our attention on the possible interaction between
SAM and the hypothalamic-hypophyseal-prolactin axis (HHPRLA). The classical scheme
for the regulation of the HHPRLA is illustrated in Fig. 2.

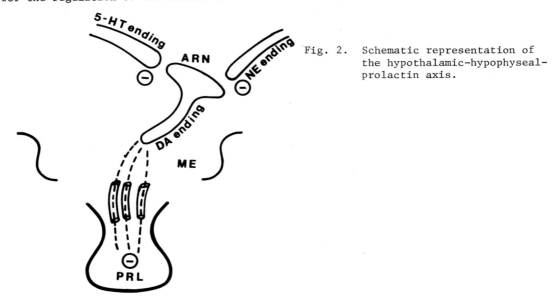

Fig. 2.   Schematic representation of
the hypothalamic-hypophyseal-
prolactin axis.

The tonic release of prolactin (PRL) is generally inhibited at the pituitary level
by prolactin-inhibiting factor (PIF) coming from the hypothalamus. Many lines of
evidence (6-II) suggest that at least the major component of PIF is dopamine (DA)
which is synthesized in the tubero-infundibular system (TIDA neurons) and released
at the level of the external layer of the median eminence (ME) into the portal blood
(12). A specific binding of DA (13) can be demonstrated at the level of the lactotropes and is associated with a constant decrease of PRL release and/or synthesis
(14-15). This inhibitory action of DA can be brought about by a number of DA mim-
etic agents which include ergot derivatives, lisuride or apomorphine. Conceivably,

DA antagonists, removing the DA tonic inhibitory tone, cause a sharp increase in PRL release both in vitro and in vivo (16-18).

Other monoamines, e.g., norepinephrine (NE), 5-HT and histamine can influence PRL secretion. However, their site of action is located at the level of the hypothalamus and not at the pituitary. It has been suggested (12) that at least in part, the stimulatory action of the central NE and 5-HT neurons on PRL release could be due to an inhibition of the activity of the TIDA neurons resulting in a decreased dopaminergic tonic inhibitory component. PRL plasma levels display in male rats a circadian pattern characterized by two peaks; the first at 4 PM and the other at 12 PM (19). The circadian regulation appears to be due predominantly to changes in the activity of 5-HT neurons (i.e., increased activity of 5-HT neurons impinging on TIDA───→decreased release of DA in the portal vessels───→increase of PRL).

In the present study we will present evidence for a possible interference of SAM on the above-mentioned regulatory components of the NEA.

Acute i.p. treatment with SAM at doses as elevated as 50 mg/kg do not modify the basal levels of PRL at any of the times examined. However, when SAM is administered chronically (5 days-last injection 1/2 hr before sacrifice) a significant and dose-dependent decrease of PRL at the 4 PM peak can be demonstrated (Fig. 3). These results induced us to further explore the possible mechanism of this inhibitory activity of SAM on PRL to determine whether or not this could be due to an interference with monoamine regulatory patterns.

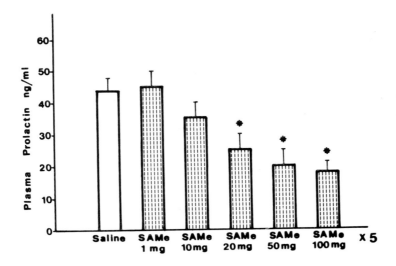

Fig. 3.   Action of a chronic treatment i.p. (5 days) with SAM at several doses on PRL plasma levels at 4 p.m.
p ⪅ 0.01

The action of SAM on the increase of PRL provoked by the powerful anti-DA benzamide
derivative sulpiride has been investigated.   Acute or chronic systemic (i.p.) administration of SAM does not appear to interfere with sulpiride-induced PRL release.
However, chronic treatment with SAM produces a significant blunting of the PRL increase evoked by the administration of TRH.   As expected the powerful DA-mimetic
compound CB-154 at the dose of 1 mg/kg completely inhibited both stimulated increases of PRL (Fig. 4).

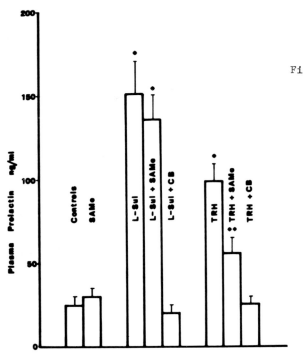

Fig. 4.   Action of chronic treatment
(5 days 50 mg/kg i.p.) with
SAM and CB 154 (1 mg/kg 6 hr
before sacrifice) on the hyper-prolactinemia induced by
L-sulpiride (0.01 mg/kg 1 hr
before sacrifice) and TRH
(50 µg/kg 2 hr before sacrifice)
p $\ll$ 0.01

When the drug is administered across the blood brain barrier (BBB) a more striking action can be observed.   In fact, as can be seen in Fig. 5, SAM administered in
the lateral ventricle 150 µg/animal 1 hr before sacrifice completely abolishes the
4 p.m. peak of PRL and inhibits the sulpiride-induced rise of the hormone.   This extremely powerful action compared to the weak activity found during peripheral administration seems to suggest that the main site of action of SAM is located across
the BBB.   Due to the rapidity of its action, a degradation of the hormone by the
induction of PCM can be ruled out.

It is tempting to speculate that SAM, when injected into the ventricular Cistern,
stimulates the activity of the TIDA neurons producing a massive release of endogenous DA which in turn is responsible for the inhibition of PRL release.

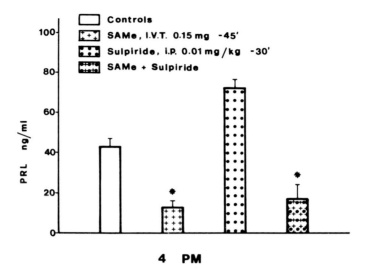

Fig. 5.  Action of an injection into the lateral ventricle of SAM
(150 µg) on PRL level at 4 p.m. with and without sulpiride
stimulation
$$p \lessapprox 0.01$$

A direct action of SAM on the lactotropes however cannot be completely excluded.  In
fact, as shown in Fig. 6, in animals in which an hyperprolactinemia is produced by
the transplantation of pituitary under the kidney followed by chronic treatment with
SAM reduces the circulating level of the hormone.  Since in this case the PRL is released from the transplanted organ separated from the hypothalamus, any inhibitory
activity found has to be related to a direct DA-mimetic action at the level of the
lactotropes.

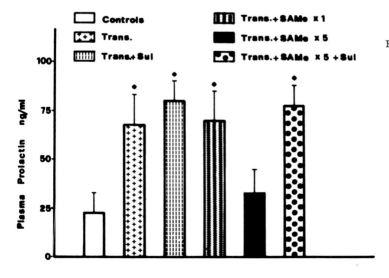

Fig. 6.  Action of acute
or chronic admin-
istration of SAM
(for details see
Fig. 4) on the
hyperprolactine-
mia induced by
pituitary implants
under the kidney
capsule.

$$p \lessapprox 0.01$$

The possibility that the treatment with SAM by activating the PCM has destroyed part of the PRL molecules, therefore decreasing the PRL circulating levels, can be excluded since an injection of sulpiride is still able to produce a maximal hyper-prolactinemia.

The action of the drug on HHPRLA appears to be even more complicated and difficult to interpret when its action is evaluated on the basis of a physiological model and not pharmacologically or surgically-induced hyperprolactinemia.  It is well known that in the afternoon of proestrus in a normal female rat a sharp rise of PRL accompanies the critical surge of LH.  As can be seen in Fig. 7, an acute injection

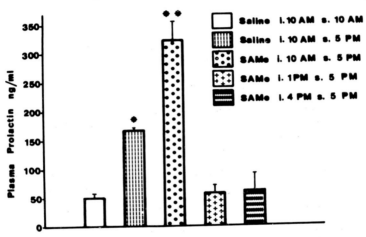

Fig. 7.    Action on PRL levels of SAM (50 mg/kg i.p.) given at different interval times from the peak at the critical period of the afternoon of the proestrus.

p $\leqslant$ 0.01

of SAM (50 mg/kg) i.p. 1 or 4.5 hr before sacrifice at the critical period, complet-ely prevents the rise of PRL.  However, when SAM is administered 7.5 hr before the peak, an opposite effect can be detected.  These puzzling results seem to suggest that the time course of the drug action is of critical importance in the regulation of the activity of the HHPRLA.

In conclusion we would like to emphasize that SAM does interfere with the HHPRLA. The modality of this interference is difficult to establish and probably has mul-tiple origins.  One of the most probable modes of action appears to be an inhibit-ion of the activity of the axis due to indirect stimulation of TIDA and/or direct DA-mimetic activity.

### REFERENCES

1.  Müller, E.E., Nistico, G. and Scapagnini, U., In: Neurotransmitters and Ante-

rior Pituitary Function, Academic Press, New York (1970).

2. Axelrod, J. and Tomchick, R., J. Biol. Chem., 233, 702 (1958).

3. Axelrod, J. and Vessel, E.S., Molec. Pharmacol., 16, 78 (1970).

4. Axelrod, J. and Weissbach, H., Science, 131, 312 (1960).

5. Kunar, M.J., Taylor, K.M. and Snyder, S.A., J. Neurochem., 18, 1515 (1971).

6. Hökfelt, T., Brain Res., 5, 121 (1967).

7. MacLeod, R.M., In: Frontiers in Neuroendocrinology, 4, Eds. L. Martini and F. Ganong, Raven Press, New York (1976).

8. MacLeod, R.M., Endocrinology, 85, 916 (1969).

9. MacLeod, R.M., Fontham, E.H. and Lehmeyer, J.E., Neuroendocrinology, 6, 283 (1970).

10. Ben-Jonathan, N., Oliver C. Mical, R.S. and Porter, J.C., Fed. Proc., Abstract No. 547 (1976).

11. Shaar, C.J. and Clemens, J.A., Endocrinology, 95, 1202 (1974).

12. Müller, E.E., Nistico, G. and Scapagnini, U., In: Neurotransmitters and Anterior Pituitary Function - Academic Press, New York, 268 (1970).

13. Cronin, M.J., Roberts, J.M. and Weiner, R.I., Endocrinology, in press, (1978).

14. Creese, I., Burt, D.R. and Snyder, S.H., Science, 192, 481 (1976).

15. MacLeod, R.M. and Kimuza, H., In: Growth Hormones and Related Peptides, Eds., G.E.W.A. Pecile and E.E. Muller, American Elsevier, New York (1976).

16. Pasteels, J.L., C.R. Acad. Sci.: D (Paris) 253, 2140 (1961).

17. Tashijan, A.H., Jr., Barowsky, N.J. and Jensen, D.K., Biochem. Biophys. Res. Commun., 43, 516 (1971).

18. Valverde, R.C., Chieffro, V. and Reichlin, S., Endocrinology, 91, 982 (1972).

19. Scapagnini, U., Gerendai, G., Clementi, L., Fiore, B. Marchetti and Prato, A., In: Environmental Endocrinology , Assenmacher and Farner, Eds., in press (1978).

# Methylation in Schizophrenia: An Old Hypothesis Revisited

## Ross J. Baldessarini[a], Giorgio Stramentinoli[b] and Joseph F. Lipinski

The Mailman Laboratories for Psychiatric Research, McLean Division of
Massachusetts General Hospital, Belmont MA 02178
and
The Department of Psychiatry, Harvard Medical School, Boston, MA

For many years, there has been considerable interest in the chemistry and pharmacology of biological transmethylation in the field of neuropsychiatry (1,2).  This
interest was largely stimulated by the fact that many natural or synthetic substances which produce a variety of psychotropic effects, including hallunications
or other reactions that also occur in psychotic illnesses, are methylated amines.
As early as 1952, Harley-Mason suggested that abnormal transmethylation of an endogenous amine, possibly dopamine, might produce a psychotomimetic compound like
mescaline.  Such products were proposed to be formed by the action of the methyl
group ($CH_3$) donor S-adenosylmethionine (SAM), a metabolite of methionine and ATP
synthesized by a specific adenosyltransferase (1).  Evidence apparently consistant
with this hypothesis was the observation that methionine, uniquely among several
amino acids, and especially when combined with an inhibitor of monoamine oxidase
(MAO), led to striking and reversible exacerbations of the psychotic symptoms of
chronic schizophrenic patients without inducing obvious signs of delirium (3,4).
It has also been reported that SAM levels in the blood of acutely psychotic (5),
but not chronically psychotic (5,6) schizophrenic subjects are low, possibly indicating its excessive utilization or deficient production (5).  Moreover, it has
been reported recently that injected SAM can exert clinically useful psychotropic
effects in depression (7).

There have also been repeated suggestions that there may be unusual methylated
phenethylamines (1,2,8) or indoleamines (1,2,9,10,11) in the urine or blood of psychotic patients.  On the other hand, the significance of these findings has been
questioned or not supported by several studies reported over the past decade.  Many
criticisms have been made of this search for unusual patterns of production or ex-

a) Recipient of NIMH career Research Scientist award MH-74370

b) Present address: Department of Biochemistry, BioResearch Co.,
   20060 Liscate (Milan), Italy

cretion of methylated metabolites on methodological grounds, particularly the use
of ambiguous analytical techniques and inadequate control of dietary and other ex-
traneous variables, as well as uncertainties regarding clinical diagnosis (see 1,2,
9-13).  Clinical studies of this kind have continued to the present time, and recent work is characterized by the use of increasingly specific biochemical methods
and greater attention to clinical variables.  These results have been both positive
(14-16) and negative (13,17-20) regarding relationships between blood levels or excretion of methylated indoleamines or phenethylamines and schizophrenia or other
severe psychiatric disorders.  The hypothesis that unusual methylated amine compounds might contribute to the pathophysiology of schizophrenia or manic-depressive
illness has been given further encouragement by reports of lower activity of MAO in
blood platelets of patients with these disorders (21).

While the possible contribution of psychoactive methylated amines to the major
idiopathic mental illnesses remains obscure, the observation that 10-40 gm loading
doses of methionine, of several amino acids, uniquely led to exacerbation of psychosis in schizophrenic patients is highly unusual among biological findings in
severe psychiatric illness in that it has been independently confirmed repeatedly
in the past decade (see 1,4,12).  The metabolic basis for this action of methionine
in schizophrenic patients, as well as the more recently reported antidepressant
action of SAM are still not understood.  While interest in the transmethylation hypothesis has waned in recent years, the fact remains that the effect of methionine
is one of the few viable clinical clues to a metabolic abnormality in psychotic
illness.  The initial suggestion that methionine might act by increasing the production of potentially psychotomimetic methylated amines by way of increased availability of SAM (22) is only partially supported by the available evidence.  Thus,
there is excellent metabolic evidence in animals, and very little in man, that the
availability of SAM is dependent on the availability of its precursor, methionine,
and on the rate of utilization of the methyl donor, which can be increased by giving
large doses of certain "methyl acceptors" (22-24).  On the other hand, the evidence
that methionine loading increases blood or tissue levels of SAM in patients remains
untested even though the means of doing so have been available for more than 10
years.  Furthermore, it remains unproven that increased availability of SAM can
increase the production of methylated biogenic amines.

These considerations have led us to reopen the study of transmethylation in animals
and man.  We were particularly interested to learn whether increased availability
of exogenous methionine can increase levels of the methyl donor SAM in human subjects.  Furthermore, we have attempted to test the prediction offered by the methylation hypothesis that increased levels of methionine and SAM in animals might increase production of methylated indoles or catechols.

## METHODS

Normal adult human subjects consented to ingesting L-methionine (Sigma Chemical Co.)
and having antecubital venous blood samples taken for assay of SAM by a sensitive
and specific radioenzymatic method (6,23), using (methyl-$^{14}$C)-SAM (New England
Nuclear Corp.).  Parallel experiments were also conducted in laboratory rats to
assess the influence of methionine on blood SAM levels, using liver as a control for
the effect of methionine on tissue levels of SAM (23,24).

In other experiments,we evaluated the effects of L-methionine, or a chemically
stable salt of SAM (Samyr, donated by BioResearch Co.), and of several other substances obtained from commercial sources in the highest available purity.  In some
of the experiments we studied the methylation of chromatographically pure (G-$^3$H)-
L-dihydroxyphenylalanine =($^3$H)-L-dopa, 10Ci/mmol, New England Nuclear Corp.) given
systemically in a tracer dose (25 µCi/200 gm rat, i.p.).  This was done by pre-
treating the rats with the powerful and irreversible MAO-inhibitor pargyline-HCl
(Eutonyl, donated by Abbott Labs.) the evening prior to giving test substances followed by ($^3$H)-L-dopa. At 5-30 min later, tissues were removed and the radioactive
metabolites were extracted; catechols and methylated metabolites were separated by
alumina column chromatography and counted by scintillation spectrometry.  These
methods have been described in detail previously (25).

In another experiment with the rat, stereotyped behavioral responses to apomorphine-
HCl (Merck; 5 mg/Kg, s.c.) were evaluated as described previously (26).  In these
experiments, pyrogallol (Sigma; 100mg/Kg, i.p.), an inhibitor of methylation (25),
was also given 30 min before apomorphine.  Similarly, L-methionine (Sigma; 500 mg/
Kg, i.p.) or SAM (BioResearch Co.; 250 mg/Kg.,i.p.) was given at 30 and 5 min before
apomorphine.  Control rats were given only saline before apomorphine.  Stereotyped
behavior was evaluated every 15 min for 2 hrs by a rating scale method (26) by an
observer unaware of the pretreatment.

In another laboratory experiment we evaluated the effect of L-methionine or SAM on
the accumulation of ($^{14}$C)-N,N-dimethyltryptamine (DMT) in lung tissue of New Zea-
land rabbits.  The animals were pretreated with the MAO inhibitor pheniprazine-HCl
(Catron, donated by Merrell National Labs.) to prevent breakdown of the labeled
indoleamines.  Later, they were given ($^{14}$C)-N-methyltryptamine (NMT, 50 Ci/mol,
donated by Dr. L.R. Mandel of Merck Institute, 9.2 µCi/rabbit) by ear vein.  Five
min later the rabbits were killed and radioactive material was extracted from the
whole lung and ($^{14}$C)-DMT was separated by a combination of silica gel thin layer
chromatography (TLC) followed by co-crystallization with authentic DMT (Sigma
Chemical Co.) and oxalic acid to constant specific radioactivity.  This method is
sensitive and highly selective for isolating DMT as its oxalate, as has been de-

scribed in detail elsewhere (27,28).

RESULTS

When methionine was given to rats by orogastric tube in a high dose (300 mg/Kg), the levels of SAM in liver increased to more than 5-fold, and remained elevated for more than 2 h (Table 1).  When parallel experiments were done with rat (Table 1) and

TABLE I.   BLOOD AND LIVER SAM LEVELS IN RAT AFTER ORAL L-METHIONINE

| Tissue | Control | L-Methionine | % of control |
|--------|---------|--------------|--------------|
| Liver | 26.6 ± 3.4 | 133.7 ± 20.9* | 514%* |
| Blood | 1.99 ± 0.25 | 2.20 ± 0.21 | 110% |

Young adult male Sprague-Dawley rats (180-220 gm) were given L-methionine (300 mg/Kg) by orogastric tube and sacrificed at 30 min later.  Controls were sacrificed without treatment at time "zero".  Data are tissue levels of SAM assayed by a radio-enzymatic method (6,23), as means ± SEM (N = 5 rats per group), in μg/g or μg/ml.

*p < 0.01 vs. controls, evaluated by Student's t-test

human subjects (Table 2), blood levels of SAM were not altered by large doses of methionine.  In the human subjects, no change was detected in whole blood, plasma, or in the cellular fractions (erythrocytes plus buffy coat) (Table 2).

TABLE II.   BLOOD LEVELS IN HUMAN SUBJECTS AFTER ORAL L-METHIONINE

SAM LEVELS (μg/ml)

| Time (min) | Whole blood | Cells | Plasma |
|------------|-------------|-------|--------|
| 0 | 0.79 ± 0.05 | 1.38 ± 0.20 | 0.17 ± 0.01 |
| 30 | 0.99 ± 0.07 | 1.38 ± 0.02 | 0.19 ± 0.01 |
| 60 | 0.84 ± 0.06 | 1.49 ± 0.24 | 0.21 ± 0.02* |

Normal adult human volunteers (2 male, 2 female, mean age = 30 years) had venous blood samples taken before, and at 30 and 60 min after a 2.5 or 10 gm oral dose of L-methionine suspended in a fruit-flavored drink.  Levels of S-adenosylmethionine (SAM) were assayed in whole or fractionated blood by a radioenzymatic method (6, 23).  For simplicity, data are presented as mean values ± SEM (N = 4  subjects); each sample assayed in triplicate; only the small rise in plasma SAM is statistically significant  (*p  0.01 by t-test).

Nevertheless, we decided to test the possible consequences of increasing levels of SAM by methionine, as this effect had been well documented in laboratory animals even at lower doses of methionine than used in the human subjects in the present work (Table 1), (1,24).  We were particularly interested in testing the prediction that increased SAM might increase the methylation of neuropharmacoligically active amines or their metabolites.  First, we reviewed the available biochemical liter-

ature to compare published values for apparent $K_m$ (half-maximal saturating concentration) for various methyl transferases of interest, with respect to the co-
substrate SAM (28-31), with normal tissue levels of SAM (1,23,28,32,33). The results
of this survey are summarized in Table 3. These results indicated that SAM levels

TABLE III.   RELATIONSHIPS OF METHYL DONOR S-ADENOSYLMETHIONINE (SAM)
WITH ENZYMES THAT METHYLATE BIOGENIC AMINES

| Enzyme | Tissue | SAM ($\mu M$) | $K_m$ (SAM) ($\mu M$) |
|--------|--------|---------------|------------------------|
| COMT | Liver | 72[a] | 14[a] |
| PNMT | Adrenal | 167[a] | 10[b] |
| HIOMT | Pineal | 127[c] | 30[c] |
| INMT | Lung | 39[a,b] | 29[b] |
|  | Brain (?)* | 46[a] | 51[a] |
| HNMT | Brain | 46[a] | 60[d] |

Enzymes (products):

    COMT:   catechol 0-methyltransferase (0-methylated catecholamines & their
          deaminated products)
    PNMT    phenylethanolamine N-methyltransferase (epinephrine)
    HIOMT:  hydroxyindole 0-methyltransferase (melatonin)
    INMT:   indoleamine-N-methyltransferase (N-methylated tryptamines)
    HNMT:   histamine N-methyltransferase (N-methylhistamine)

Species:     a   rat
                b   rabbit
                c   beef
                d   guinea pig

These data are means of published values (28-31).

*Presence of INMT in brain remains controversial as many assays of its putative
activity are based on methods later found to be unreliable (see 28).

are normally in excess of the $K_m$ for SAM with methyltransferase enzymes in several
tissues, although for COMT, INMT and HNMT, endogenous SAM in rodent tissues was
relatively close to $K_m$. This observation suggested that these enzymes might normally be less nearly saturated with methyl donor, and so more easily "pushed" by
increasing tissue levels of SAM.

This prediction was first tested with a representative catechol substrate for COMT,
($^3$H)-L-dopa. We found that even huge doses of L-methionine had little effect on
the ratio of methylated-to free-catechol metabolites of labeled dopa recovered from
brain or viscera (heart, liver and kidney tissue) of the rat (Table 4). In a small
number of other experiments, we also found that large doses of exogenous SAM had
little effect on the methylation of ($^3$H)-L-dopa in the mouse (data not shown), al-

though the mouse was found to methylate dopa so rapidly (about 30% in 5 min and more than 90% within 15-30 min in brain and viscera) as to make the expected finding of increased methylation difficult to observe. In the rat, there was a suggestion that the highest dose of methionine given (1000 mg/kg) may even have slightly de-creased the ratio of methylated-to catechol-metabolites of dopa (Table 4). Further-more, exogenous S-adenosylhomocysteine (SAH) produced a clear dose-dependent in-hibition of methylation (Table 4).

TABLE IV. EFFECT OF METHIONINE AND OTHER AGENTS OF METHYLATION OF ($^3$H)-L-DOPA

| Treatment | Dose (mg/kg) | Methylated: Catechol Metabolites (% of control) | | |
|---|---|---|---|---|
| | | Brain | Viscera | control) |
| L-methionine | 500 | 85.0 ± 5.4 | 87.8 ± 3.9 | |
| | 1000 | 82.8 ± 3.9* | 78.5 ± 3.8* | |
| S-adenosylhomo-cysteine | 10 | 115.5 ±10.0 | 95.7 ±10.0 | |
| | 100 | 84.9 ± 2.3* | 46.6 ± 2.3** | |
| Nicotinamide | 1000 | 102.0 ± 9.8 | 122.0 ±12.4 | |
| Guanidineacetic Acid | 100 | 103.4 ± 4.3 | 89.3 ± 5.3 | |
| | 200/d x 4 | 101.7 ± 6.6 | 100.0 ± 8.7 | |

Male Sprague-Dawley rats (180-220 gm) were pretreated with the MAO inhibitor pargy-line (100 mg/kg, i.p.) 16-18 hr before the experimental treatments at the doses in-dicated to limit the metabolites formed to those of dopa and its amine products. Thirty min later rats were given ($^3$H)-L-dopa (25 μCi, i.p.), and 15 or 30 min after giving this tracer, brain and pooled viscera tissues (whole heart and kidneys and approximately 1 gm of liver) were removed to ice, homogenized in perchloric acid, and 0-methylated vs. catechol metabolites were separated by alumina column chroma-tography, all as described in detail previously (25). To compensate for potential artifactual changes in uptake of the tracer into some tissues (notably, the known competition of methionine and dopa for entry into the brain (1), data were computed as ratios of tritium radioactivity in the two fractions (methylated vs. free cate-chols) rather than as absolute quantities of the metabolites. The data are pre-sended here for convenience as percent of control values (means ± SEM) for groups of 9-10 rats.

* p < 0.05

** p < 0.01

In the same series of experiments we also evaluated the potential of large doses of substances proposed (1) as potentially clinically useful inhibitors of methylation of ($^3$H)-L-dopa. In these experiments, large doses of nicotinamide or guanidine-acetic acid had little effect (Table 4). In a similar experiment, the methylatable catechol-estrogen estradiol (100 mg/Kg) had no effect on the methylation of dopa (±5% of control).

Pyrogallol, an inhibitor of COMT had a profound apomorphine-potentiating and duration-prolonging effect on stereotyped behavior in the rat (Table 5). In contrast, methionine and SAM in large doses had no antagonistic or duration-reducing effect in this behavioral paradigm (Table 5).

TABLE V.   EFFECT OF METHYLATION ON THE BEHAVIORAL ACTIONS OF APOMORPHINE

| Condition (N) | Mean sterotypy score $\pm$ SEM | % of Control |
|---|---|---|
| Control (22) | 13.1 $\pm$ 0.5 | 100 |
| Pyrogallol (100 mg/kg) (6) | 22.8 $\pm$ 0.6 | 174 * |
| L-Methionine (500 + 500 mg/kg) (12) | 134.4 $\pm$ 0.9 | 102 |
| SAM (250 + 250 mg/kg) (6) | 12.2 $\pm$ 1.0 | 93 |

The drugs were given intraperitoneally to N rats 30 min prior to the subcutaneous injection of the catechol-containing central dopamine receptor agonist apomorphine-HCl (5.0 mg/kg). The doses of L-methionine and SAM were also repeated at 5 min prior to the apomorphine. Control animals vary significantly and so were pooled from several experiments. Stereotyped behavior was evaluated by a "blind" observer with a rating-scale technique (26). Data are mean behavioral scores, as totals of individual values obtained each 15 min for 2 hrs. The effect of pyrogallol, an inhibitor of catechol-0-methyltransferase capable of depleting endogenous SAM (25), was to increase the maximal response of apomorphine and to prolong its action by 15 min, presumably by preventing its inactivation by methylation. Methionine and SAM were without effect.

* $p < 0.001$ by t-test

Since endogenous SAM levels are unusually close to its $K_m$ for rabbit lung INMT (Table 3), and since DMT-formation bears a particularly interesting hypothetical relationship to psychosis (2,10,11), we also evaluated the effects of methionine and SAM on the methylation of NMT, the immediate precursor of DMT. In these experiments, rather than an increase in DMT-production, we found a striking decrease in newly synthesized labeled DMT recovered from rabbit lung by a reliable and sensitive method (Table 6).

DISCUSSION

Our present results (Table 1) have confirmed the observation (22-24) that large doses of methionine lead to increased production of the methyl donor SAM sufficiently in excess of its utilization as to increase its tissue concentrations. Since human blood is reported to contain activity of the SAM-synthesizing enzyme, methionine-adenosyltransferase, in both erythrocytes and leukocytes (34,35), it was somewhat surprising to find that large doses of methionine had little or no effect on SAM levels in any blood fraction in human subjects. The doses used (2.5 or 10

TABLE VI.   EFFECT OF METHIONINE OR SAM TREATMENT ON ($^{14}$C)-DMT
            ACCUMULATION

| Treatment | Control | Methionine | SAM |
|---|---|---|---|
| ($^{14}$C)-DMT | 725 ± 76 | 269 ± 70* | 302 ± 70* |
| (pCi/gm lung) | | | |
| Per Cent of Control | 100% | 40%* | 44%* |

Rabbits were pretreated with an MAO inhibitor (pheniprazine, 10 mg/kg, i.p., 6 hr
earlier) and L-methionine or S-adenosylmethionine (SAM) (100 mg/kg, s.c.) 30 min
before i.v. injection of ($^{14}$C)-N-methyltryptamine (donated by D. L. Mandel, Merck
Institute).  Animals were killed 4 min later and ($^{14}$C)-N-N-dimethyltryptamine (DMT)
was selectively recovered from extracts of lung by a highly specific chromatographic
cocrystallization method.  Further data and a detailed discussion of the methods
used have been presented elsewhere (28).

* p ∠ 0.02 vs. controls by Student's t-test; data are mean values ± SEM for 3
  rabbits per condition.

gm) were somewhat below those reported to induce transient worsening of psychosis
in schizophrenics (generally 10-20gm), but in excess (over 100mg/kg) of doses previously found to raise tissue levels of SAM in laboratory animals (24).  In addition,
even a very large dose of methionine (300 mg/kg), while increasing liver SAM levels
over 5-fold, had only a small effect (25% increase) on SAM in whole blood of the
rat (Table 1).  This small increase in blood may represent a "spill-over" of SAM
formed in other tissues such as liver.  Since the kinetics of methionine-adenosyltransferase recovered from blood have evidently not yet been evaluated, especially
with respect to a possible excess of normal blood concentrations of methionine or
of limiting concentrations of ATP, the explanation of this observation is not clear.
An unfortunate practical clinical consequence, however, is that the prediction remains unproved that methionine would increase tissue SAM levels in man as it does
in animals in most tissues, including brain (1,22-24), except blood (Table 1).  In
addition we had hoped to evaluate further the interesting observation by Andreoli
and Maffei (5) that blood SAM levels are decreased in acute phases of schizophrenia,
but not different from normal in chronic schizophrenics (5,6).  This might have
been done by measuring rates of change of blood SAM after giving sub-psychotogenic
doses of methionine to normal and acutely psychotic subjects to assess possible
differences in rates of formation and utilization of SAM.  But since human blood
SAM levels are unresponsive even to 10 gm of methionine (Table 2), this strategy
cannot be followed.  It is also important to note that even 10 gm doses of meth-

ionine, while producing very mild light-headedness or nausea, had no grossly
detectable psychotropic effects in normal human subjects, as we had expected based
on prior tests of this question (1).

When we evaluated changes in the methylation of L-dopa (Table 4) or of NMT (Table
6) after large doses of methionine or SAM, there was little or no increase in the
recovery of methylated metabolites of dopa or of DMT, respectively. We also found
(Table 5) that methionine and SAM had no effect on the potency or duration of action
of apomorphine in the production of stereotyped gnawing in the rat. In contrast,
pyrogallol, an inhibitor of COMT, clearly potentiated this catechol-alkaloid (Table
5). All cf these results are consistent with the few available data that fail to
indicate increased production of methylated metabolites in man after large doses of
methionine (See 1; Table 7), including a recent study of DMT excretion that was

TABLE VII.   SUMMARY OF ATTEMPTS TO DEMONSTRATE EFFECTS OF METHIONINE
             ON METHYLATION IN HUMAN SUBJECTS

| Metabolites Assayed | Methionine Dose (gm/day) | Result | Reference |
|---|---|---|---|
| VMA[a] | up to 40 (also gave tryptophan) | little effect | Berlet et.al., 1965 (45) |
| MN, NMN | ca.20 (also gave MAO inhibitor) | no effect | Kakimoto et al., 1967 (46) |
| VMA, MHPG | up to 20 | no effect | Antun et al., 1971 (47) |
| HVA, VMA, etc. | up to 10 | no effect | Coper et al., 1972 (48) |
| DMT, NMT | up to 4 | no effect[b] | Oon et al., 1977 (20) |

These results summarize the experience re urinary methylated metabolites in normal
or schizophrenic human subjects using adequate analytic methods.

Abbreviations:   DMT,    N, N-dimethyltryptamine
                 HVA,    homovanillic acid
                 MHPG,   3-methoxy-4-hydroxy-phenylethyleneglycol
                 MN,     metanephrine
                 NMN,    normetanephrine
                 NMT,    N-methyltryptamine
                 VMA,    vanillylmandelic acid

a (methionine may have interfered with the VMA assay)
b (results inconclusive; 1 patient given rel. small dose of methionine)

performed with careful methods (20). We also studied the production of DMT in rabbit lung as it is one of the few tissues that almost certainly contains INMT (27,
28). In this experiment levels of newly synthesized labeled DMT in lung tissue un-
expectedly appeared to be _decreased_ by large doses of exogenous methionine or SAM
(Table 6). The latter effect may reflect the repeatedly demonstrated ability of
the metabolite SAH to inhibit methyltransferases (including lung INMT) in competition with SAM _in vitro_ (29-31,36). It has also been reported that methionine can
increase tissue levels of SAH in liver (3) and brain (37). Our present results with
the methylation of ($^3$H)-L-dopa appear to be the first _in vivo_ observation consistent
with an inhibition of methylation by SAH (Table 4). The treatment of patients with
this metabolite or with structural analogs of it has recently been suggested as a
possible experimental treatment of psychotic patients, based on the methylation
hypothesis (36).

Several facts about the regulation of methyltransferase reactions consistent with
our generally negative results in Tables 4,5 and 6 are now becoming clearer. First,
most methyltransferases that use catechols or indoles as substrates appear to have
SAM requirements ($K_m$) that are _below_ resting tissue levels of SAM in most tissues
(Table 3). Second, not only is SAH an effective competitive end-product inhibitor
of most methyl transfer reactions utilizing its precursor, SAM, but there is even
evidence that some methylated metabolites themselves exert similar inhibitory effects. This effect has recently been demonstrated with DMT, using rabbit lung INMT
(36), although it is not clear whether other methyltransferases are subject to similar regulation by their methylated products. Thus it is unlikely that increases
of SAM by methionine or exogenously administered SAM would increase the production
of methylated metabolites by such well-regulated enzymes that already have adequate
amounts of the methyl donor under normal conditions.

One other observation that arises from the present experiments is that two "methyl
acceptor" molecules, nicotinamide and guanidineacetic acid (1) had little effect on
the methylation of L-dopa, even when given in high or repeated doses (Table 4). The
result with nicotinamide is thus consistent with our previous observations of a lack
of effect of large doses of nicotinamide on tissue levels of SAM in the rat, in
contrast to other more toxic methylatable substances (1,22). This lack of effect
thus fails to support the idea that large doses of nicotinamide might be a useful
treatment of schizophrenic patients based on its ability to inhibit the methylation
of biogenic amines (38) - a "mega-vitamin" therapeutic effect for which there is
now virtually no scientifically compelling evidence (1,2,39,40). Similarly, guanidineacetic acid, which is converted to the biologically apparently almost inert

metabolite creatine, has been suggested by Dr. S. Matthysse as a potential methyl-ation-inhibiting therapy in schizophrenia (1). It has been given safely in the past in large doses (several gm/day) to patients with poliomyelitis (41). But a-gain, our results (Table 4) fail to support an appreciable anti-methylation effect of guanidine-acetic acid.

In conclusion, the present results fail to support the predictions of the methyl-ation hypothesis that increased tissue levels of SAM produced by large doses of L-methionine (or of SAM itself) would increase the production of methylated metabo-lites of catechols or indoles, and notably, of DMT. The question remains of how methionine exerts its consistent psychosis-worsening effect in schizophrenics. The present results are not consistent with the hypothesis that psychotogenic methyl-ated catechol or indole products of SAM are responsible. Possibly other metabolic pathways than those considered here are involved, such as the production of homo-cysteine (1,42). Methionine is known to have toxic metabolic effects (43), espec-ially on the liver (44), and it has been found to have behavioral effects in the rat that seem to be unrelated to its role as a methyl donor (42). While the pre-sent results seem to indicate the implausibility of the methylation hypothesis, the effect of methionine in schizophrenia remains a valid clinical phenomenon, one of the few viable leads to a metabolic abnormality in schizophrenia and still wor-thy of further study.

## SUMMARY

Large doses of L-methionine were found to have no behavioral effects in normal human volunteers, and failed to increase blood concentrations of SAM, the main methyl donor in most methyltransferase reactions. Similarly, methionine had little effect on SAM levels in rat blood, while increasing these levels in the liver more than 5-fold. As a model for the study of methylation of catechols, the ratio of methylated: catechol metabolites of ($^3$H)-L-dopa recovered from rodent brain and viscera was evaluated. Methionine or exogenous SAM in very high doses had almost no effect on the methylation of this catechol, and various "methyl acceptor" mole-cules, including nicotinamide, guanidineacetic acid, and estradiol similarly had little effect. In another model of catechol O-methylation, high doses of methio-nine or SAM had no effect on the behavioral actions of the catechol-aporphine apo-morphine in the rat. In the rabbit, methionine and SAM not only failed to increase the production of DMT in lung, but actually decreased it, possibly in part due to end-product inhibition induced by SAH, which strongly inhibited the methylation of L-dopa in the rat in vivo. These results fail to support several predictions of the

138     R. J. Baldessarini, G. Stramentinoli and J. F. Lipinski

"methylation hypothesis" concerning the pathophysiology and potential treatment of idiopathic psychotic disorders. and leave the consistent clinical worsening effects of methionine in schizophrenia unexplained.

ACKNOWLEDGEMENTS

This work has been partially supported by U.S. Public Health Science (NIMH) research grants MH-25525 and MH-16674, and an award from the Scottish Rite (NMJ of USA) Schizophrenia Foundation.  Based in part on papers submitted to the Archives of General Psychiatry and the Journal of Neurochemistry, March, 1978.

REFERENCES

1.  Baldessarini, R.J., Int. Rev. Neurobiol., 18, 41 (1975).

2.  Gillin, J.C., Stoff, D.M. and Wyatt, R.J., In: Psychopharmacology: A Generation of Progress, Lipton, M.A., DiMascio, A. and Killam, K.F., (Eds.), Raven Press, New York, 1097 (1978).

3.  Pollin, W., Cardon, P.V., Jr., and Kety, S.S., Science, 133, 104 (1961).

4.  Cohen, S., Nichols, A., Wyatt, R. and Pollin, W., Biol. Psychiatry, 8, 209 (1974).

5.  Andreoli, V.M. and Maffei, F., Lancet, ii, 922  (1975).

6.  Matthysse, S. and Baldessarini, R.J., Amer. J. Psychiatry, 128, 1310 (1972).

7.  Agnoli, A., Andrioli, V., Casacchia, M. and Cerbo, R., J. Psychiatric Res., 13, 43 (1976).

8.  Friedhoff, A.J. and Van Winkle, E., Nature, 194, 897 (1962).

9.  Rosengarten, H. and Friedhoff, A.J., Schizophrenia Bull., 2, 90 (1976).

10.  Editorial, Lancet ii, 140 (1974).

11.  Gillin, J.C., Kaplan, J., Stillman, R. and Wyatt, R.J., Amer. J. Psychiatry, 133, 203 (1976).

12.  Wyatt, R.J., Termini, B.A. and Davis, J.M., Schizophrenia Bull., 4, 10 (1971).

13.  Carpenter, W.T., Fink, E.B., Narasimhachari, N. and Himwich, H.E., Amer. J. Psychiatry, 132, 1067 (1975).

14.  Narasimhachari, N. and Himwich, H.E., Biochem. Biophys. Res. Commun., 55, 1064 (1973).

15.  Cottrell, A.C., McLeod, M.F. and McLeod, W.R., Amer. J. Psychiatry, 134, 322 (1977).

16.  Friedhoff, A.J., Park, S., Schweitzer, J.W., et al., Biol. Psychiatry, 12, 643 (1977).

17. Wyatt, R.J., Mandel, L.R., Ahn, H.S., et. al., Psychopharmacologia, 31, 265 (1973).

18. Lipinski, J.F., Mandel, L.R., Ahn, H.S., et al., Biol. Psychiatry, 9, 89 (1974).

19. Angrist, B., Gershon, S., Sathananthan, G., et al., Psychopharmacology, 42, 29 (1976).

20. Oon, M.C., Murray, R.M., Rodnight, R., et al., Psychopharmacology, 547, 171 (1977).

21. Wyatt, R.J., Potkin, S.G., Gillin, J.C. and Murphy, D.L., In: Psychopharmacology: A Generation of Progress, Lipton, M.A., DiMascio, A. and Killam, K.F., (Eds.), Raven Press, New York, 1083 (1978).

22. Baldessarini, R.J., In: Amines and Schizophrenia, Himwich, H.E., Kety, S.S. and Smythies, J.R. (Eds.), Pergamon Press, Oxford, 199 (1967).

23. Baldessarini, R.J. and Kopin, I.J., J. Neurochem., 13, 769 (1966).

24. Baldessarini, R.J., Biochem. Pharmacol., 15, 741 (1966).

25. Baldessarini, R.J. and Greiner, E., Biochem. Pharmacol., 22, 247 (1973).

26. Tarsy, D. and Baldessarini, R.J., Neuropharmacology, 13, 927 (1974).

27. Walker, R.W., Ahn, H.S., Mandel, L.R. and Vanden Heuvel, W.J.A., Analyt. Biochem., 47, 228 (1972).

28. Stramentinoli, F. and Baldessarini, R.J., J. Neurochem., 1978, in press.

29. Deguchi, T. and Barchas, J., J. Biol. Chem., 246, 3175 (1971).

30. Baudry, M., Chast, F. and Schwartz, J.C., J. Neurochem., 20, 13 (1973).

31. Saavedra, J.M., Coyle, J.T. and Axelrod, J., J. Neurochem., 20, 743 (1973).

32. Eloranta, T. O., Biochem. J., 166, 521 (1977).

33. Stramentinoli, G., Gualano, M., Catto, E. and Algeri, S., J. Gerontology, 32, 392 (1977).

34. Baldessarini, R.J. and Bell, W.R., Nature, 209, 78 (1966).

35. Dunner, D.L., Cohn, C.K., Weinshilboum, R.M. and Wyatt, R.J., Biol. Psychiatry, 6, 215 (1973).

36. Domino, E.F., Arch. Int. Pharmacodyn. Ther., 221, 75 (1976).

37. Schatz, R.A., Vunnum, C.R. and Sellinger, O.Z., Neurochem. Res., 2, 27 (1977).

38. Hoffer, A. and Osmond, H., Acta Psychiat. Scand., 40, 171 (1964).

39. Matthysse, S. and Lipinski, J.F., Ann. Rev. Med., 26, 551 (1975).

40. Ban, T.A., Lehmann, H.E. and Deutsch, M., Comm. Psychopharmacol., 1, 119 (1977).

41. Fallis, B.D. and Lam, R.L., J.A.M.A., 150, 851 (1952).

42. Beaton, J.M., Smythies, J.R. and Bradley, R.J., Biol. Psychiatry, lo, 45 (1975).

43. Park, L.C., Baldessarini, R.J. and Kety, S.S., Arch. Gen. Psychiatry, 12, 346 (1965).

44. Hardwick, D.F., Applegarth, D.A., Crockcroft, D.M., et al., Metabolism, 19, 381 (1970).

45. Berlet, H.H., Matsumoto, K., Pscheidt, G.R., et al., Arch. Gen. Psychiatry, 13, 521 (1965).

46. Kakimoto, Y., Sano, I., Kanazawa, A., et al., Nature, 216, 1110 (1967).

47. Antun, F.T., Burnett, G.B., Cooper, A.J., et al., The effects of L-methionine (without MAOI) in schizophrenia. J. Psychiatric Res., 8, 63 (1971).

48. Coper, H., Deyhle, G., Fahndrich, G., et al., Pharmakopsychiat. Neuro-psycho-pharmakol., (Stuttgart) 5, 177 (1972).

# Antidepressant Effects of Adenosyl-methionine: Clinical and Methodological Issues Emerging from Preliminary Trials

**D. Kemali, M. Del Vecchio, L. Vacca, A. Amati, L. A. Famiglietti and T. Celani**

Department of Psychiatry, Ist Medical School, University of Naples, Naples, Italy

The hypothesis that depression is due to a metabolic disorder involving catecholamines, serotonin or, most likely, their functional balance, prompted the use of various therapeutic agents. On the other hand, the introduction of psychoactive drugs into the treatment of depressive states has stimulated both clinical and basic biological research.

A large number of antidepressant drugs, belonging to different categories, are at present available. All of them possess, to different extent, a depression-relieving effect, a psychomotor-activating effect, and an anxiolytic effect.

The compounds most widely used by clinicians belong to the group of tricyclic (imipramine, amitriptyline and derivatives) and tetracyclic (maprotiline) MAO inhibitors, besides lithium salts and some recently developed molecules such as nomifensine and viloxazine, as well as some serotonin precursors (tryptophan). These compounds induce an appreciable antidepressant response, but nevertheless their marked side effects are frequently unbearable, especially by outpatients. Another problem is related to the therapy-resistant depressions which bring many aspects of depression research into sharper focus.

The use of S-adenosylmethionine (SAM) in the treatment of depressed patients has been recently made possible through the availability of this molecule in a stable form. SAM is one of the main methyl donors in the central nervous system (CNS) and other tissues (1); it is involved in most transmethylation processes. SAM participates in the metabolism of biogenic amines in the CNS and its cerebral level can be modified by the use of common antidepressant drugs (2,3). Furthermore, it has been observed that depressed-patients have reduced catechol 0-methyltransferase (COMT) activity in red cells (4). This might indicate a decrease of the concentration of the methyl donor, SAM.

In view of this, preliminary clinical trials on the use of SAM in the treatment of depressed patients are of peculiar interest. The results evaluated according to the Hamilton Rating Scale for Depression (HRS) (5) indicated that the patients improved when treated with SAM (6,7,8,9,10). In our department, 28 depressed patients scor-

ing more than 30 in the HRS, entered a single-blind trial of SAM versus chlorimipramine (11).   The patients were divided in two groups, (A and B), each formed at
random.   According to Kielholz nosological criteria, they were diagnosed as follows:
<u>Reactive depression</u>, 12 patients; <u>Neurotic depression</u>, 8 patients; <u>Somatogenic de-</u>
<u>pression</u>, 3 patients; <u>Endogenous depression</u>, 5 patients.

Group A received 150 mg of SAM <u>pro die</u> for three weeks divided into two administrations, injected slowly i.v., whereas Group B was given 100 mg of chlorimipramine
<u>pro die</u> following the same procedure.   Clinical evaluations were performed before
the treatment and once a week during the trial.   HRS total scores obtained at the
beginning, after 7 days and at the end of the trial were evaluated by means of
Student's t-test, which showed significant variations induced by the treatment in
both groups (Tab. 1).

Table 1.   <u>HRS scores for patients treated with SAM and chlorimipramine (see text)</u>

|  | | Mean values | Standard deviation | Student t-test* | |
|---|---|---|---|---|---|
|  | | | | t | p |
| A) | SAM treatment | | | | |
|  | before treatment | 38.43 | ±6.69 | | |
|  | after 7 days | 33.43 | ±7.75 | 4.6771 | <0.0001 |
|  | at the end of treatment | 30.07 | ±6.94 | 5.759 | <0.0001 |
| B) | Chlorimipramine treatment | | | | |
|  | before treatment | 36.14 | ±6.24 | | |
|  | after treatment | 31.79 | ±3.49 | 3.6094 | <0.005 |
|  | at the end of treatment | 26.64 | ±2.71 | 6.3802 | <0.001 |

*compared with values before the treatment

Focusing attention on items Nos. 1 (depressive mood), 2 (guilt), 3 (suicidal tend-
encies), 7 ( work and interests), 8 (retardation), which are the most representative
of the "depressive core" of HRS, 46% of the patients on SAM and 30% of patients on
chlorimipramine improved after 7 days of treatment.   Percentages at the end were
60% and 74%, respectively (see Table 2).

Table 2.   <u>Percentage of improvements in relation to the items 1-2-3-7 and 8 of HRS</u>
<u>total score after 7 days and at the end of the treatment with antidepres-</u>
<u>sant drugs (see 11) under conditions reported in Table 1.</u>

|  | SAM treatment | Chlorimipramine treatment |
|---|---|---|
| After 7 days | 46% | 30% |
| At the end of treatment | 60% | 74% |

After 7 days $\chi^2$ gives significant value between the percentage of the two groups whereas at the end of the treatment the difference is not significant ($\chi^2$= 0.983; p = N.S.). These results indicate that SAM exerts a more rapid action, but chlorimipramine is as effective after 3 weeks.

Besides clinical investigations, quantitative analysis of bioelectric activity of the brain should be performed when a compound which is supposed to possess psychotropic properties is administrated (12). Our data relevant to this effect (13) have been collected from the EEG recordings of 18 patients treated with SAM. Table 3 shows statistical evaluation of the differences in the right and left hemisphere in 5 single bands of cerebral electric activity. Quantitative analysis of delta, theta, alpha and beta frequency bands have been done in temporal and occipital leads in both cerebral hemispheres. Tau value - indicated by T- is constantly lower than the value of standard reference, indicated by (T). Since the differences are not significant, it may be assumed that SAM, within the limits of this procedure, does not affect EEG variables (see Table 3).

Table 3.  Effects of SAM treatment on EEG frequency bands in depressed patients (see 14)

|        |       | $\overline{X}d$ | Sd | T | (T) |
|--------|-------|------|------|---------|-------|
| delta  | Right | 0.48 | 4.5 | 0.6315 | 2.034 |
|        | Left  | 0.06 | 7.7 | 0.045 | 2.036 |
| theta  | Right | 0.001 | 3.00 | 0.00196 | 2.034 |
|        | Left  | 0.09 | 3.9 | 0.134 | 2.036 |
| alpha  | Right | 1.15 | 7.7 | 0.871 | 2.034 |
|        | Left  | 0.63 | 7.5 | 0.488 | 2.036 |
| beta 1 | Right | 0.0057 | -- | -- | -- |
|        | Left  | 0.34 | 4.08 | 0.485 | 2.036 |
| beta 2 | Right | 0.97 | 5.1 | 0.979 | 2.038 |
|        | Left  | 0.97 | 3.8 | 1.763 | 2.038 |

n  =  18

$\overline{X}d$  =  Mean of differences (before/during treatment)

Sd  =  Mean squared discard of differences

T  =  Actual tau coefficient

(T) =  Standard tau coefficient

--  =  Very low differences, not calculated

$\alpha$  =  0.05

Unfortunately, a small number of clinical trials has been performed; only the study by Scarzella (10) and our own evaluate effects of SAM vs. chlorimipramine. Preliminary data indicate that SAM exerts an antidepressant effect which is detectable after the first week. Moreover, no side effect has been observed except for occasional and mild symptoms of anxiety.

On the whole, the present results are encouraging but not completely satisfactory. We think that further clinical research may result in more reliable results, provided that a more comprehensive strategy of investigation could be established.

In this connection, a proposed methodology should consider that the clinical assessment has to be performed according to multiaxial classificatory criteria (14), and the variations of symptomatology have to be recorded according to specific rating scales exploring depressive symptoms, i.e., HRS, Quantitative Depression Inventory (QDI), Zung Self-Rating Scale.

Monitoring of SAM blood levels should be performed so as to obtain information on the relationship between the dose and the effect of the drug.

Moreover, computerized EEG (CEEG) spectral analysis may show a substantial contribution in discriminatory variations of electric cerebral activity as an index of the brain functional organization. Fig. 1 gives an explanatory demonstration of CEEG spectral analysis we are performing in depressed patients treated with SAM. A detailed description of the CEEG analysis that our group uses has been published by Kemali et al. (15) .

The figures show the following:
First line: Spectra of frequencies from 0.5 to 32 c/s of frontal $(A_2F_4)$, parietal $(A_2C_4)$ and occipital $(A_2O_2)$ leads in right hemisphere.
Fourth line: Spectra of frequencies from 0.5 to 32 c/s of symmetric leads in the left hemisphere $(A_1F_3; A_1C_3; A_1O_1)$.
Second line: Coherence between the frequencies in the right and left leads.
Third line: The dashed line gives the values of the phase concordance between the frequencies in the right and left leads. Frequency bands are represented on the abscissa and the power of signals on the ordinates, e.g., in cell graphics (see Fig. 1). Furthermore, in the power spectra (first and fourth line) several parameters for each peak are calculated (relative activity, baricentric frequency).

This methodology allows a very accurate study of each single band of frequency and is more sensitive than simple frequency analysis.

Table 4 shows, e.g., the same EEG spectral parameter changes, particularly in the beta band, after treatment with SAM.

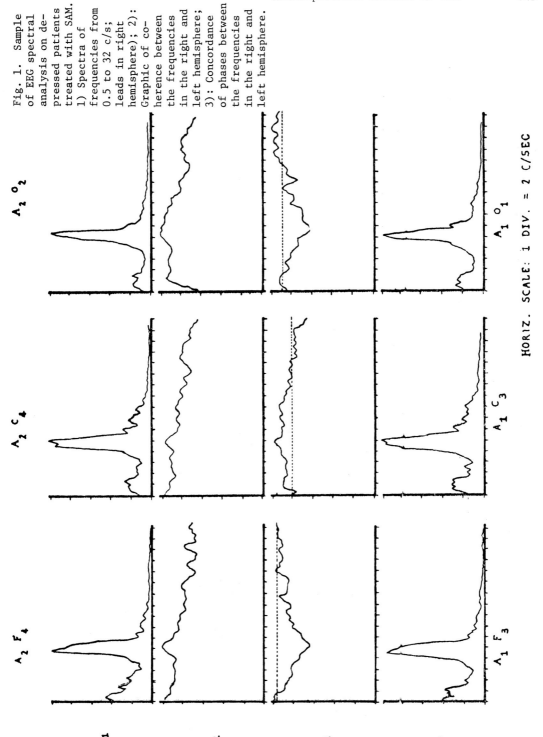

Fig. 1. Sample of EEG spectral analysis on depressed patients treated with SAM. 1) Spectra of frequencies from 0.5 to 32 c/s; leads in right hemisphere); 2): Graphic of coherence between the frequencies in the right and left hemisphere; 3): Concordance of phases between the frequencies in the right and left hemisphere.

HORIZ. SCALE: 1 DIV. = 2 C/SEC

     D. Kemali *et al.*

TABLE 4     <u>SPECTRAL EEG VARIATIONS IN 4 DEPRESSED PATIENTS</u>
                <u>AFTER TREATMENT WITH SAM</u>

| | $\delta$ | $\vartheta$ | $\alpha$ | $\beta$ |
|---|---|---|---|---|
| Relative Activity | / | < | > | / |
| Baricentric Frequency | / | / | / | < |
| Baricentric Radius | / | / | / | < |

The Greek letters indicate the EEG frequency bands.

">" indicates that the spectral parameter is higher after treatment

"<" indicates the opposite

"/" indicates no relevant variations

Work is in progress in our laboratory with the following objective: clinical evalua-
tions are scheduled for long intervals to collect a pool of data correlating blood
levels of SAM and CEEG recording.

In conclusion, it is our opinion that a large number of clinical trials will have
to be carried out with identical methodology, in order to ascertain both the antidepressant effect of SAM and possible neurophysiological variations produced by
this therapy.

### REFERENCES

1. Axelrod, J., in <u>The Biochemistry of Adenosylmethionine</u>, Salvatore, F., Borek, E.,
   Zappia, V., Williams-Ashman, H.G. and Schlenk, F. Eds., Columbia University
   Press, New York, 53º (1977).

2. Iversen, L.L., in <u>Frontiers in Catecholamine Research</u>, Usdin, E. and Snyder, S.,
   Eds., Pergamon Press, 403 (1973).

3. Jarrott, B., in <u>Frontiers in Catecholamine Research</u>, Usdin, E. and Snyder, S.,
   Eds., Pergamon Press, 113 (1973).

4. Cohen, C.K., Dunner, D., Axelrod, J., <u>Science</u>, 170, 1323 (1970).

5. Hamilton, M.J., <u>Neurol. Neurosurg. Psychiat.</u>, 23, 56 (1960).

6.  Fazio, C., Andreoli, V., Agnoli, A., Casacchia, M., Cerbo, R., Min. Med., 64, 1515 (1973).

7.  Agnoli, A., Fazio, C., Andreoli, D., De Carolis, V., Bonamini, F., Casacchia, M., Cerbo, R., Ruggiero, D., Carolei, A., Clin. Terap., 1, 13 (1975).

8.  Mantero, M., Pastorino, P., Carolei, A., Agnoli, A., Min. Med., 66, 4098 (1975).

9.  Agnoli, A., Andreoli, V., Casacchia, M., Cerbo, R., J. Psychiat. Res., 13, 43 (1976).

10. Scarzella, R., VI World Congress of Psychiatry, Honolulu, Commun. (1977).

11. Del Vecchio, M., Iorio, G., Cocorullo, M., Vacca, L., Amati, A., VI World Congress of Psychiatry, Honolulu, Commun. (1977).

12. Fink, M., Ann. Rev. Pharmacol., 9, 241 (1969).

13. Celani, T., Iorio, G., Vacca, L., Amati, A., Del Vecchio, M., Curr. Therap. Res., 23, 225 (1978).

14. Ottosson, G.D., Perris, G., Psychol. Med., 3, 238 (1973).

15. Kemali, D., Vacca, L., Marciano, F., Nolfe, G., Celani, T., Iorio, D., Atti XXXIII Congresso Nazionale Soc. Ital. Psychiat., 265 (1977).

# Adenosylmethionine and Chronic Ammonia Intoxication

**Gianni Benzi**

Istituto di Farmacologia, Facolta di Scienze, Universita di Pavia, Pavia, Italia

## INTRODUCTION

Under the conditions of ammonia detoxication during hyperammonemia syndromes, the ammonium-glutamate system is the most closely involved. Even though the basic event is the amidation of glutamate to glutamine (1), it should be pointed out that all the participants in the ammonium-glutamate system are involved in the detoxication process (2,3,4). On the other hand, some participants in the ammonium-detoxicating system (e.g., pyruvate, $\alpha$-ketoglutarate, oxaloacetate) are closely connected both with glycolysis and with the tricarboxylic acids cycle. In the study of relationships between hyperammonemia and energy transduction, it has been demonstrated that, in the acute syndrome, ammonium ions are able to increase the cerebral Gibbs free energy (4,5) and that ammonia intoxication is always accompanied by an increase in the lactate:pyruvate and $NADH:NAD^+$ cytoplasmic ratios in the brain (6). Other findings (7,8), suggest a direct interference of ammonium ions on energy production mechanisms.

Based on the role of ammonium ions on brain energy transduction (2,3,4,5,9), a study was carried out in the rat on the cerebral effect of experimental chronic hyperammonemia induced by 3 different daily doses of ammonium acetate, as well as on the influence exerted by the simultaneous daily treatment with some participants in the biological system of S-adenosyl-L-methionine (SAM): methionine (as a precursor), S-adenosyl-L-methionine (as activated substance), adenosine (as breakdown product). The interference of SAM with cerebral processes of energy transduction (4) and its well-known importance in transmethylation and trans-sulfuration processes (10,11), suggest its potential role in hyper-ammonemia syndromes. Its activity is assumed also because the final product of its biological transformation, cisteine, conjugates with $\alpha$-ketoglutarate to give mercaptopyruvate and glutamate, the key intermediate of the ammonium-glutamate detoxication system.

In order to evaluate at cerebral level both the effect of the chronic administration of ammonium acetate, and the possible interference of the participants in the SAM

149

system, the behavior of indicative cerebral enzymatic activities on the homogenate in toto and/or on the crude mitochondrial fraction was investigated. The enzymes studied were: lactate dehydrogenase (1-lactate: $NAD^+$ oxidoreductase, EC 1.1.1.27) for the glycolytic pathway; citrate synthase (citrate oxaloacetate-lyase, EC 4.1.3. 7) and malate dehydrogenase (1-matate:$NAD^+$ oxidoreductase, EC 1.1.1.37) for the Krebs' cycle; total NADH-cytochrome c reductase (NADH-cytochrome c oxidoreductase, EC 1.6.99.3) and cytochrome oxidase (ferrocytochrome c: oxygen oxidoreductase, EC 1.9.3.1) for the electron transport chain.

## MATERIALS AND METHODS

Sprague-Dawley female rats (initial weight $100 \pm 8$ g) kept under standard caging conditions (temperature: $22 \pm 1^{\circ}C$, relative humidity $60 \pm 5\%$; lighting cycle: 12 hr light and 12 hr darkness; low noise disturbance) and fed a standard pellet diet with water ad libitum were used. All animals used for the experiments were treated with ammonium acetate or sacrificed for the preparation of subcellular fractions between 9:30 and 10:30 a.m.

At the beginning of treatment, 80 animals were selected at random and subdivided into three lots of 5 groups each: 1 control group and 4 groups administered daily, 6 days a week, high doses of ammonium acetate i.p. for 40 days. Three of these 4 groups were simultaneously treated i.m. with equimolar doses of SAM, methionine or adenosine. The doses chosen corresponded to highly active ones, commonly employed in experimental investigations. On the whole, the animals employed were subdivided as follows: lot 1 - 1 group of control animals (group C, 10 rats) given saline solu — tion i.p. and 4 groups of animals treated i.p. for a total of 40 days (6 days a week) with 33 mg/kg of ammonium acetate (1 daily administration: 9:30-10:30 a.m.) not preceded (group $A_1$, 5 rats) or preceded by pretreatment and subsequent i.m. treatment (2 daily administrations: 8:00-9:00 a.m. and 4:00-5:00 p.m.) with equi- molar doses of SAM (20 mg/kg, group $B_1$, 5 rats), methionine (7.5 mg/kg, group $D_1$, 5 rats) and adenosine (13.5 mg/kg, group $E_1$, 5 rats). Lot 2 = 4 groups of animals treated i.p. for a total of 40 days (6 days a week) with 100 mg/kg of ammonium ace- tate (1 daily administration: 9:30-10:30 a.m.) not preceded (group $A_2$, 5 rats) or preceded by pretreatment and subsequent i.m. treatment (2 daily administrations: 8:00-9:00 a.m. and 4:00-5:00 p.m.) with equimolar doses of SAM (group $B_2$, 5 rats), methionine (group $D_2$, 5 rats) and adenosine (group $E_2$, 5 rats) as above; lot 3 = 4 groups of animals treated i.p. for a total of 40 days (6 days a week) with 300 mg/kg of ammonium acetate (1 daily administration: 9:30-10:30 a.m.) not preceded (group $A_3$, 5 rats) or preceded by pretreatment and subsequent treatment i.m. (2 daily administrations: 8:00-9:00 a.m. and 4:00-5:00 p.m.) of the above mentioned equimolar doses of SAM (group $B_3$, 5 rats), methionine (group $D_3$, 5 rats) and adenosine (group $E_3$, 5 rats).

At the end of the treatment period, the animals were sacrificed by decapitation (9:30-10:30 a.m.) and their brains removed within 15 sec in a precooled box at $-5\,^{\circ}C$. The tissue was then immediately immersed into, and washed with, a cold sucrose solution, 0.32 M. The brains were then weighed and homogenized in sucrose (0.32 M) for 10 sec in a Potter-Elvehjem homogenizer with only two strokes (up and down) of a teflon pestle (total clearance = 0.25 mm). The homogenate thus obtained was then diluted (10% w/v) and an aliquot of each sample was taken for the evaluation of enzymatic activities on the homogenate in toto. The remaining homogenate was centrifuged (Sorvall RC-5 Supercentrifuge) for the preparation of the crude mitochondrial fraction (12) and the protein content was evaluated (13). On both the homogenate and mitochondrial preparation samples, the following enzymatic activities were measured: malate dehydrogenase (14), total NADH-cytochrome c reductase (15), cytochrome oxidase (16,17). In homogenate samples the activity of lactate dehydrogenase was also evaluated (18), while the activity of citrate synthase was measured in the mitochondrial preparation samples (19). Calculations of enzymatic activities were performed using the straight portion of the reaction curves obtained through the graphic recording of extinction variations (Beckman model 25 spectrophotometer). The results were expressed as specific activities ($\mu$moles.min$^{-1}$.mg protein$^{-1}$, and statistically analyzed with the Student's $\underline{t}$ test.

### RESULTS

Table 1 shows the values of enzymatic activities (homogenate and mitochondrial fraction) found after the chronic administration of ammonium acetate at the dose of 33 mg/kg i.p. Some groups of animals (B1, D1 and E1) were simultaneously submitted to two daily administrations of equimolar doses of SAM, methionine or adenosine. It can be seen that the chronic administration of ammonium acetate was not responsible for any significant change in the hyaloplasmic and mitochondrial enzymatic activities studied (comparison C-$A_1$). Also the i.m. treatment with the various substances participating in the SAM system (methionine, SAM, adenosine) caused no significant modifications (comparisons $A_1$-$B_1$; $A_1$-$D_1$; $A_1$-$E_1$).

Table 2 reports the values of enzymatic activities (homogenate and mitochondrial fraction) following the chronic administration of ammonium acetate at the dose of 100 mg/kg i.p. In this case, a decrease in some enzymatic activities can be observed, (i.e., of malate dehydrogenase, as evaluated on the homogenate) and of total NADH-cytochrome c reductase, as evaluated both on the homogenate in toto and on the mitochondrial fraction (comparison C-A2). The i.m. treatment with the participants in the SAM system (comparisons $A_2$-$B_2$; $A_2$-$D_2$; $A_2$-$E_2$) did not prove able to prevent the hyperammonemia-induced decay of the enzymatic activities described

TABLE I.  CEREBRAL ENZYMATIC ACTIVITIES RELATED TO THE ENERGY TRANSDUCTION

Effect of the treatment with S-adenosyl-L-methionine, methionine or adenosine on the chronic administration of ammonium acetate (33 mg/kg i.p.).

| Groups of rats | | Homogenate | | | | Mitochondria | | | |
|---|---|---|---|---|---|---|---|---|---|
| | | Lactate dehydrogenase | Malate dehydrogenase | Total NADH cytochrome c reductase | Cytochrome oxidase | Citrate synthase | Malate dehydrogenase | Total NADH cytochrome c reductase | Cytochrome oxidase |
| Controls | 0 | 0.544 ± 0.035 | 1.36 ± 0.06 | 0.032 ± 0.001 | 0.219 ± 0.020 | 0.037 ± 0.003 | 0.801 ± 0.051 | 0.053 ± 0.002 | 0.374 ± 0.039 |
| Treated with: ammonium acetate | $A_1$ | 0.617 ± 0.060 | 1.23 ± 0.14 | 0.028 ± 0.003 | 0.184 ± 0.027 | 0.031 ± 0.002 | 0.804 ± 0.057 | 0.045 ± 0.007 | 0.327 ± 0.038 |
| Idem plus SAM | $B_1$ | 0.626 ± 0.0.8 | 1.20 ± 0.03 | 0.028 ± 0.002 | 0.205 ± 0.027 | 0.034 ± 0.003 | 0.858 ± 0.029 | 0.042 ± 0.003 | 0.394 ± 0.045 |
| Idem plus Methionine | $D_1$ | 0.596 ± 0.035 | 1.17 ± 0.04 | 0.024 ± 0.001 | 0.159 ± 0.012 | 0.034 ± 0.004 | 0.798 ± 0.040 | 0.040 ± 0.004 | 0.374 ± 0.038 |
| Idem plus Adenosine | $E_1$ | 0.632 ± 0.027 | 1.28 ± 0.13 | 0.028 ± 0.002 | 0.199 ± 0.021 | 0.038 ± 0.002 | 0.929 ± 0.059 | 0.048 ± 0.001 | 0.343 ± 0.069 |

Statistical analysis: C or $B_1$ or $D_1$ or $E_1$ versus $A_1$ = p 0.05 (t Student test) in any case.

The enzymatic activities ($\mu$moles.min$^{-1}$.mg protein-1) were evaluated in homogenate and in crude mitochondrial fraction from rat brain (mean values ± S.E.M.: N = 10, for control rats; N = 5, for each group of treated rats).

TABLE II. CEREBRAL ENZYMATIC ACTIVITIES RELATED TO ENERGY TRANSDUCTION

Effect of the treatment with S-adenosyl-L-methionine, methionine or adenosine on the chronic administration of ammonium acetate (100 mg/kg i.p.).

| Groups of rats | | Homogenate | | | | Mitochondria | | | |
|---|---|---|---|---|---|---|---|---|---|
| | | Lactate dehydro-genase | Malate dehydro-genase | Total NADH cytochrome c reductase | Cytochrome oxidase | Citrate synthase | Malate dehydro-genase | Total NADH cytochrome c reductase | Cytochrome oxidase |
| Controls | C | 0.544 $\pm$0.035 | 1.36 $\pm$0.06 | 0.032 $\pm$0.001 | 0.219 $\pm$0.020 | 0.037 $\pm$0.003 | 0.801 $\pm$0.051 | 0.053 $\pm$0.002 | 0.374 $\pm$0.039 |
| Treated with: ammonium acetate | $A_2$ | 0.612 $\pm$0.011 | 1.12 $\pm$0.05 | 0.026 $\pm$0.001 | 0.184 $\pm$0.017 | 0.035 $\pm$0.001 | 0.824 $\pm$0.060 | 0.042 $\pm$0.001 | 0.365 $\pm$0.039 |
| Idem plus SAM | $B_2$ | 0.601 $\pm$0.043 | 1.11 $\pm$0.06 | 0.026 $\pm$0.002 | 0.223 $\pm$0.042 | 0.037 $\pm$0.003 | 0.891 $\pm$0.065 | 0.045 $\pm$0.004 | 0.394 $\pm$0.056 |
| Idem plus Methionine | $D_2$ | 0.602 $\pm$0.036 | 1.15 $\pm$0.07 | 0.027 $\pm$0.002 | 0.193 $\pm$0.010 | 0.035 $\pm$0.001 | 0.828 $\pm$0.029 | 0.041 $\pm$0.002 | 0.402 $\pm$0.029 |
| Idem plus Adenosine | $E_2$ | 0.582 $\pm$0.057 | 1.28 $\pm$0.10 | 0.029 $\pm$0.003 | 0.221 $\pm$0.040 | 0.026 $\pm$0.004 | 0.710 $\pm$0.055 | 0.040 $\pm$0.004 | 0.361 $\pm$0.045 |
| Statistical analysis: values of P (t Student test) | | | | | | | | | |
| $A_2$ versus C | | >0.05 | <0.05 | <0.01 | >0.05 | >0.05 | >0.05 | <0.01 | >0.05 |
| $B_2$,$D_2$ or $E_2$ versus $A_2$ | | >0.05 | >0.05 | >0.05 | >0.05 | >0.05 | >0.05 | >0.05 | >0.05 |

The enzymatic activities ($\mu$moles·min$^{-1}$·mg protein$^{-1}$) were evaluated in homogenate and in crude mitochondrial fraction from rat brain (mean $\pm$ S.E.M.: N = 10, for control rats; N = 5, for each group of treated rats).

TABLE III.    CEREBRAL ENZYMATIC ACTIVITIES RELATED TO ENERGY TRANSDUCTION

Effect of the treatment with S-adenosyl-L-methionine, methionine or adenosine on the chronic administration of ammonium acetate (300 mg/kg i.p.).

| Groups of rats | Homogenate | | | | Mitochondria | | | |
|---|---|---|---|---|---|---|---|---|
| | Lactate dehydro- genase | Malate dehydro- genase | Total NADH cytochrome c reductase | Cytochrome oxidase | Citrate synthase | Malate dehydro- genase | Total NADH cytochrome c reductase | Cytochrome oxidase |
| Controls          C | 0.544 $\pm$0.035 | 1.36 $\pm$0.06 | 0.032 $\pm$0.001 | 0.219 $\pm$0.020 | 0.037 $\pm$0.003 | 0.801 $\pm$0.051 | 0.053 $\pm$0.002 | 0.374 $\pm$0.039 |
| Treated with: ammonium acetate A$_3$ | 0.602 $\pm$0.030 | 1.22 $\pm$0.06 | 0.028 $\pm$0.003 | 0.182 $\pm$0.023 | 0.040 $\pm$0.003 | 0.782 $\pm$0.093 | 0.045 $\pm$0.003 | 0.354 $\pm$0.059 |
| Idem plus SAM    B$_3$ | 0.603 $\pm$0.034 | 1.22 $\pm$0.09 | 0.029 $\pm$0.004 | 0.182 $\pm$0.029 | 0.042 $\pm$0.004 | 0.788 $\pm$0.073 | 0.045 $\pm$0.004 | 0.316 $\pm$0.049 |
| Idem plus methionine    D$_3$ | 0.598 $\pm$0.051 | 1.21 $\pm$0.10 | 0.027 $\pm$0.002 | 0.213 $\pm$0.047 | 0.032 $\pm$0.001 | 0.658 $\pm$0.064 | 0.037 $\pm$0.002 | 0.323 $\pm$0.002 |
| Idem plus adenosine    E$_3$ | 0.525 $\pm$0.016 | 1.21 $\pm$0.07 | 0.028 $\pm$0.001 | 0.198 $\pm$0.040 | 0.039 $\pm$0.004 | 0.702 $\pm$0.074 | 0.041 $\pm$0.001 | 0.340 $\pm$0.058 |
| Statistical analysis: values of P (t Student test) | | | | | | | | |
| C,B$_3$ or D$_3$ versus A$_3$ | >0.05 | >0.05 | >0.05 | >0.05 | >0.05 | >0.05 | >0.05 | >0.05 |
| E$_3$ versus A$_3$ | <0.01 | >0.05 | >0.05 | >0.05 | >0.05 | >0.05 | >0.05 | >0.05 |

The enzymatic activities ($\mu$moles.min$^{-1}$.mg protein$^{-1}$) were evaluated in homogenate and in crude mitochondrial fraction from rat brain (mean $\pm$ S.E.M.: N = 10, for control rats; N = 5, for each group of treated rats).

above.

Table 3 shows the values of enzymatic activities (homogenate and mitochondrial fraction) following the chronic administration of ammonium acetate at the dose of 300 mg/kg i.p. The results obtained demonstrate that no enzymatic activities were significantly changed with regard to the syndrome (comparison $C-A_3$) or as a consequence of treatment with the participants in the SAM system (comparisons $A_3-B_3$; $A_3-D_3$; $A_3-E_3$), except for lactate dehydrogenase (comparison ($A_3-E_3$).

## DISCUSSION

Of the three doses of ammonium acetate administered daily for 40 days, only the medium one (100 mg/kg) caused a moderate decrease in two cerebral enzymatic activities related to energy transduction (malate dehydrogenase; NADH-cytochrome c reductase). This raises the problem of understanding why a threefold dose (300 mg/kg) did not cause any significant modification, at least in the cerebral enzymatic activities affected by the 100 mg/kg dose. One might hypothesize that ammonia metabolism could take place adequately with the lowest dose (30 mg/kg) and that only the highest dose of ammonium acetate administered "intraperitoneally" is capable of potentiating the hepatic and tissue metabolism of ammonium ions by drug-induction mechanisms. The non-intervention of this last mechanism might account for the slight cerebral enzymatic derangement caused by 100 mg/kg of ammonium acetate.

At any rate, chronic treatment with ammonium acetate exerts a moderate effect on the cerebral enzymatic activities involved in energy transduction. Indeed, lactate dehydrogenase, citrate synthase, and cytochrome oxidase are never affected, nor is mitochondrial malate dehydrogenase. The total NADH-cytochrome c reductase is decreased, both in the homogenate and in the motochondrial fraction, malate dehydrogenase being decreased only in the homogenate. This finding can be related to the multilocular distribution of these enzymes. On the whole, however, our date are in agreement with the experimental observation (20) that during acute or gradual hyperammonemia no significant changes can be found in some cerebral enzymatic activities related to energy and ammonium-detoxication metabolisms, e.g., $Na^+-K^+$-ATPase, pyruvate kynase, glutamate dehydrogenase, glutamine synthase.

It is also interesting that no significant effects were observed with the simultaneous administration of equimolar doses of some participants in the SAM biological system (methionine, SAM, adenosine), particularly with regard to the moderate decrease of enzymatic activities induced by the chronic treatment with 100 mg/kg/day i.p. of ammonium acetate. With regard to an acute cerebral hyperammonemia syndrome induced by ammonium acetate, the continuous intracarotid perfusion of a very high dose of SAM to the dog (4) further increased the turnover of ammonia and the change of Gibbs free energy, and made the resting transmembrane potential more strongly positive (increased cerebral excitability). The date obtained in this investigation apparently indicate that a possible interaction between the ammonium-detoxicating system and SAM system might take place indirectly, at cerebral level, through a tissular change of biological intermediates, rather than by direct enzymatic activation, at least as far as cerebral enzymes related to energy release, such as those studied by us, are concerned. This finding should on the other hand be related to the already mentioned poor tendency of the hyperammonemia syndrome to affect the cerebral enzymatic activities connected with energy metabolism (present data) and ammonium-detoxicating metabolism (20).

ACKNOWLEDGEMENTS

We thank Mrs. M.L. Riva for assistance in the preparation of the manuscript and Mrs. G. Garlaschi for technical assistance.

REFERENCES

1.  Weil-Malherbe, H., in Neurochemistry, Eds. Elliot, K.A., Page, I.H. and Quastel, J.H., 321 (1962).

2.  Benjamin, A.M. and Quastel, J.H., Biochem. J., 128, 631 (1972).

3.  Benjamin, A.M. and Quastel, J.H., J. Neurochem., 25, 197 (1975).

4.  Benzi, G., Arrigoni, E., Strada P., Pastoris, O., Villa, R.F. and Agnoli, A., Biochem. Farmac., 26, 2397 (1977).

5.  Hawkins, R.A., Miller, A.L., Nielsen, R.C. and Veech, R.L., Biochem. J., 134, 1001 (1973).

6.  Hindfelt, B. and Siesjö, B.K., Scand. J. Clin. Lab. Invest., 28, 365 (1971).

7.  McKhann, G.M. and Tower, D.B., Am. J. Physiol., 200, 420 (1961).

8.  Worcel, A. and Erecinska, M., Biochim. Biophys. Acta, 65, 27 (1962).

9.  Schenker, S., McCandless, D.W., Brophy, E. and Lewis, M.S., J. Clin. Invest., 46, 838 (1967)

10. Greenberg, D.M., Adv. Enzymol., 25, 395 (1963).

11. Lombardini, J.B. and Talalay, P., Adv. Enz. Regul., 9, 349 (1971).

12. De Robertis, E., Pellegrino De Iraldi, A., Rodrigues De Lores Arnaiz, G. and Salganicoff, L., J. Neurochem., 9, 23 (1962).

13. Lowry, O.H., Rosebrough, N.J., Farr, A.L. and Randall, R.J., J. Biol. Chem., 193, 265 (1951).

14. Ochoa, S. in Methods in Enzymology, Eds. Colowick, S.P. and Kaplan, N.O., Academic Press, New York, 1, 735 (1955).

15. Nason, A. and Vasington, F.D., in Methods in Enzymology, Eds. Colowick, S.P. and Kaplan, N.O., Academic Press, New York, 6, 409 (1963).

16. Smith, L., in <u>Methods of Biochemical Analysis</u>, Ed. Glick, D., Wiley-Interscience, 2, 427 (1965).

17. Wharton, D.C. and Tzagoloff, A., in <u>Methods in Enzymology</u>, Eds. Estabrook, R.W. and Pullman, M.E., Academic Press, New York, 10, 245 (1977).

18. Bergmeyer, H.U. and Bernt, E., in <u>Methods in Enzymatic Analysis</u>, Ed. Bergmeyer, H.U., Academic Press, New York, 2, 574 (1976).

19. Sudgen, P.H. and Newsholme, E.A., <u>Biochem. J.</u>, 150, 105 (1975).

20. Rooney, E. and O'Donovan, D.J., <u>Biochem. Pharmac.</u>, 24, 1995 (1975).

# Subject Index

# Author Index